alive!

alive!

lifestyle changes to age-proof your mind and body

RACHNA CHHACHHI

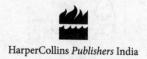

HarperCollins *Publishers* India

First published by HarperCollins *Publishers* in 2021
A-75, Sector 57, Noida, Uttar Pradesh 201301, India
www.harpercollins.co.in

2 4 6 8 10 9 7 5 3 1

P-ISBN: 978-93-9035-189-3
E-ISBN: 978-93-9035-190-9

Typeset in 11/14.8 Adobe Caslon Pro at
Manipal Technologies Limited, Manipal

Printed and bound at
Replika Press Pvt. Ltd.

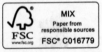

This book is produced from independently certified FSC® paper to ensure
responsible forest management.

To Mama

They say I look like you
I wish you could see
We discuss the songs you love each night
And I smell your fragrance next to me
Wherever you are, Mama
I know you're smiling down at me
Coz when I look into the mirror
I see you in me

RIP 13 November 2020

Contents

Part 3: The Body

Part 4: The Learnings

Part 5: The New Order

Preface

The voices from the world are growing.

*L*aurence works for a bank in Paris and is getting no menopausal symptoms at age 53 even though her periods are scanty. She won't deny herself dessert immediately after dinner.

Aradhna is 23, a French Wine scholar (FWS), who rejected work at a fancy five-star hotel as a sommelier and chose to teach yin yoga instead. A job does not fit into her grand scheme of things.

Ronnie lives in New Delhi. At 81, he loves his whisky and eats non-vegetarian food every day. He has no health issues.

At age 37, Andrew is already a well-known change leader. His daily practice to keep himself mentally fit is meditation and riding his mountain bike in the forest.

Steven lives in the Greater Boston area. At 79, his brain is sharp and agile, and if he doesn't agree with you, prepare for a long-drawn-out discussion where you can't beat him because of his depth of knowledge. He enjoys his red wine every evening.

Camille travelled from France to India to learn yoga. She is just 26 and feels that it is her generation that is going to popularize sustainable living.

Chhachhi Sir, as everyone calls him, is 91. In Gurgaon, his mid-morning cup of coffee has a dollop of Baileys Irish Cream and he gets irritated if he doesn't get his second helping on time. He has never had a lifestyle or any other disease.

These people are not following a lifestyle propagated by health gurus or experts. They are carving their own path. And through this book, we are going to learn what they are doing right despite embracing habits that are seen as unhealthy.

Why did I interview these people across the world?

As a health expert, I saw them live a life that was contradictory to the tenets and advice given by every nutritional health expert on how to live a long and disease-free life. I was seeking answers because they were not following the 'guidelines' to be as healthy as they were. As CALM as they are.

So, I reached out to the universe to give me the answers. I interviewed over fifty people across the world for this book. Over the years, I have treated and guided thousands of others who have rediscovered good health by beating a chronic disease. All of them come from different parts of the world, with different genetic make-ups, blood groups, lineages and upbringing. They don't necessarily follow what health and nutritional guidelines insist upon to 'stay healthy'—a lot of what I practice and preach isn't what you see on Dr Google or nutritional talks on social media. And yet, the people I treat are living examples of good health and are ageing well with a wonderful quality of life. The fifty people I spoke to were doing the same, but not under any guidance. It was like they had an intuitive sense about it.

What were they doing right?

Everything that is written in this book will leave you in a good mood and feeling positive. Every story has the purpose of helping you leave your toxicity behind so you can consistently enjoy the journey of life, every day, day after day. And the habits cultivated by the people featured in this book are supported by science.

This book is about a new beginning where shifting your energy brings about a change in your immune system.

For each one of us who have been short-changing ourselves and pretending to live while we rush from one activity to another, this book will help you hit the pause button, reflect on how you can make your every day more meaningful in a structured manner, and put the joy of the everyday back into your life. Once this joy is back, it impacts everything around you—your health, family, relationships, work, quality of life and your longevity. I coined a saying that goes, 'Leaf your life back.' Since you can't take back your life, you can do it one leaf at a time, until the 'tree' that is you starts to grow again, this time with denser leaves, a cooler shade and stronger roots.

Enjoy, imbibe, and follow, whether you are age 20, 30, 40, 60, or 80. The book is packed with clinical research data quoted in the references section, so you will know that every aspect of the lifestyle that I have recommended has scientific and anecdotal proof in the form of the inspirational journeys shared. Walk with me, a little briskly, while I take you on the journey of being alive while you live.

It's not about the years; it's about what you put in the years.

Why Steve?

I have never met him in person, but he is an old friend.

Steven P. Cohen (I call him Steve) is an author and thought leader who lives in the Greater Boston area. After law school, he spent twelve years in politics and with the government in the US. The next twelve years he worked in his family's business. Each of these activities required lots of negotiation. When most people would be making retirement plans, Steve launched The Negotiations Skills Company, and ran it for twenty-five years. Simultaneously, he was a professor at Groupe HEC (Paris) and Brandeis University's International Business School (Boston). He has coached companies and employees across the world, including the Tatas and the Aditya Birla Group in India.

Steve has authored *Negotiating Skills for Managers* (McGraw-Hill [and Tata McGraw-Hill], 2002) and *The Practical Negotiator: How to Argue Your Point, Plead Your Case, and Prevail in Any Situation* (Career Press, October 2013).

I 'met' him twenty years ago, when he was 59 years old and I was running a gender practices company. He was the 'negotiation' king, so I sought his advice to help women advocate for themselves in the workplace. I literally cold-called him and he responded almost immediately. That was in 2000. He wrote a regular column for us online (my entire business model was online even then). Later, I had to shut down my company, but Steve and I kept in touch via email. I remember sending him an extremely emotional email after the 2008 Mumbai terror attacks, and his response was warm and reassuring.

From 59 to his current age of 79, when the quality of life often declines, Steve remains a poster boy for good health, me time, and mental agility. I have seen his journey from a senior executive coach helping people change habits and perspectives to leading a supposedly semi-retired life.

He remains active in companies where he sits on the board and as trustee of his community foundation. He gardens, and proudly sends pictures of his six-year-old grandson meditating.

When he sent me that serene picture of his grandson, I was reminded of what the Dalai Lama had once said, 'If every eight-year-old in the world is taught meditation, we will eliminate violence from the world within one generation.'

As a global consultant, his professional knowledge, and exposure to various societies, cultures and organizations, gives Steve a unique perspective and quirky sense of humour that makes him relatable, warm and easy to learn from. He has provided solutions for a broad range of negotiating challenges faced by people across dozens of countries. Each question/problem was submitted by a real person looking for advice.

The one thing that struck me about Steve is his integral being is not just limited to what he does professionally. Almost every conversation with him has a mention of Andréa, his wonderful spouse, his children and now grandchildren, his gardening and his glass of red wine. All this while we discuss work, the world, politics, visiting each other. Steve is a complete person and wears that on his sleeve. For each one of you trying to make excuses for not being able to find time to be healthy, Steve's professional success and genial personality will make you sit up and say, 'If he can, so can I.'

Over to Steve.

Foreword

About twenty years ago I was surprised to receive an invitation from an unknown person in India. Rachna Chhachhi was a little bit ahead of the curve; she had founded *Redforwomen*, an online community for women struggling to get back to the workplace or become entrepreneurs after a maternity break. This was well before such activities were commonplace. Rachna wanted me to become the dotcom's advice columnist/agony aunt.

It was an intriguing idea, but I was not sure about being the right fit. I had never been to India (then) nor had I ever been a woman. Nonetheless, the opportunity was appealing. I wrote responses to a large number of fascinating questions from women throughout India.

With Rachna's permission, I started carrying the advice column on my US-based website. Before long, I was getting queries about an even broader range of questions from all over the world. Several years later, a collection of those questions and answers was published as *The Practical Negotiator*.

Rachna Chhachhi is a remarkable person. Her ability to combine very old and very new ideas—about communicating, healthy bodies, good nutrition—makes her a significant contributor to the well-being of the people lucky enough to get to know her. This book represents one culmination of her visionary, yet practical, approach.

While we've never met, our conversations are the broad-ranging kind, like old friends have.

When she invited me to contribute to this book it was clear Rachna is interested in how people can make good choices as they age. Folks want to live long lives, but unless that length is accompanied by well-being and continuing mental engagement, long can be a drag. With this compendium of insights into herself and the world around her, Rachna's book will help you make a better life for yourself. As a holistic nutrition expert whose practice spans twenty-seven countries, Rachna holds together her patients, clients and two hundred-plus coaches with the same ease as she holds together her rebuilt health. After having suffered a major health crisis that would have left most defeated, she began her mission to help others.

This book is part of that mission. It will help you lead a healthier, happier life. If only you follow it.

May 2020   Steven P. Cohen

Introduction
Dr Taruna Madan Gupta

This book is focused on understanding the connection between our immune system and our mind and therefore, the power and responsibility we have towards our own health and happiness. If you tell a layperson that if they are healthy, they will be happier, they may not understand the connection. But through this book, Rachna has systematically shown how bad moods are linked to a lack of physical and emotional balance, dysregulated immunity and nutritional deficiencies.

As a scientist and immunologist, I have not only seen this implemented in Rachna's work, but also seen the clinical aspects of how her treatment impacts the quality of life. Though inflammation is a creative, healing process of our immune response, persistent or chronic inflammation eats away our resources and deprives us of any stored resources for emergencies such as an infection. The connection between inflammation and disease is well established but what is not acknowledged is that when we restore immune homeostasis, we are reducing the risk of diseases and getting a better quality of life and longevity as a result.

Of course, for the layperson reading this book, this connection may seem oblique. But when you look at the clinical data, which is what I'm trained to look at, there is large acceptance for inflammation reduction leading to a lower risk of diseases in the entire medical community. From that perspective, the methodology listed by the author is supported by various therapeutic strategies in practice today for chronic ailments. The focus of the treatment is to either reduce inflammation or suppress immune response so that the symptoms of the disease can be reduced. Medications are to save lives in critical conditions though with long-term usage their risk-benefit ratio becomes lopsided. Tinkering with the immune response comes with its own drawbacks. The need of the hour is to restore the immune homeostasis and the holistic healing with meditation, yoga and nutrition can help you achieve it without side effects, and that is the beauty of this kind of healing.

I will share an example, as a scientist, to help you understand the above.

Cardiovascular disease involves inflammation of the blood vessels, making the heart do more work and on top of it, gets reduced nutrition and oxygen. When this inflammation is reduced with medications or surgery, the heart gets healthier. Medications can reduce high blood pressure, high cholesterol and triglycerides, all of which harden the arteries, hence reducing blood flow to and from the heart. Nutrition is naturally stored as cholesterol or fat and is the seed for genesis of hormones. Therefore, these medications can raise the risk of type 2 diabetes, and very often end up killing the natural flora and probiotics present in the digestive tract. Killing of natural flora in the gut has been linked to dysregulated immunity and higher inflammation levels. So, the same drugs that help the heart patient stabilize, can also cause problems which now need attention not only from cardiologists, but also from diabetologists, gastroenterologists and very often, psychiatrists, to help the patient get the quality of life he or she deserves.

But when the heart is made healthier through an anti-inflammatory lifestyle that also reduces the bad lipids and high blood pressure, the good side effect of that lifestyle is that it increases the gut flora and natural probiotics. By default, a heart healthy diet reduces anxiety levels. This leads to a rejuvenated immune system ready to face challenges. Hence, the second option, which has been clinically proven. Rachna has quoted Dr Dean Ornish in her book on how he, as a cardiologist, has provided clinical evidences for the second option for the last thirty years, hence demonstrating that a healthier heart which does not require a bypass surgery can be achieved with minimal or no medication or surgery.

I have been working on clinical research related to infectious pathogens including the COVID-19 virus and one thing is very well-accepted by the entire medical fraternity— you are prone to develop severe infections if your immune system is suppressed. The immune system is suppressed by specific immunosuppressive drugs, for example, that are used for acceptance of a transplant or in autoimmune patients. There are also individuals with lifestyle ailments like cardiovascular disease, type 2 diabetes and older people on the list of those who are immunocompromised.

The first thing that compromises immunity is high levels of stress and every person's response to the same stress may be different. This fact is not very well known to the layperson and the author has emphasized and quoted clinical data on the power of the mind to reduce stress levels, increase good quality sleep and also given techniques to do the same. Very often, we fail to understand that fifty per cent of our stress, anxiety and low immunity can repair itself with eight hours of sleep. Hundreds of sleep studies have proven this. Most of the times, the solutions are simpler than we thought.

When you look at the human cells, the basic unit of life, as I do—in a lab—a few things become very clear. One of the most powerful of these is that we are meant to repair—*vis medicatrix naturae*—a phrase attributed to the father of medicine, Hippocrates, which means that when organisms are left alone, they have a natural ability to heal themselves. Of course, we all know that there are certain extremes that form exceptions to this rule. Beyond these extremes, there is no such thing as the damage being done and the body not working overtime to repair it. Presence of stem cells in every organ and tissue of the body are strong evidences towards our body's ability to heal. Increased inflammation in itself is a response of our immune system to help us repair. But when we do not heed and support our mind and body to repair, chronic diseases set in. As a scientist involved in clinical research, I personally believe in strengthening the natural repair mechanisms of our body and mind. This book is about helping you understand how to help yourself so that the medical treatments will be much more effective with minimal side effects. And who knows, you may not need medical treatment if you follow the advice given in the book diligently.

Dr Gupta, MPharm, PhD is Scientist F and Head, Innate Immunity, National Institute for Research in Reproductive Health (ICMR), Mumbai.

Part 1

The Truth

When too many people around us die, at an age and time they were not meant to, it's time to review the ugly truth.

1

The Apathy of Good Health

At least once a week, I get to hear of how someone I know personally or through work suddenly succumbed to death. Last week, a childhood friend was found by the police in his apartment. He was only 46 and had had a sudden heart attack. Over the last couple of years, I have lost many friends, colleagues, acquaintances; more than a dozen of my classmates are no more. All of them were the class of 1987.

And yet, there are people who are doing something right, without even realizing it. We will learn from their engaging life stories and habits. There is something spiritual about the way they live, but it has nothing to do with religion. It is like a deep prayer, but only to the self. We will also realize, as we read ahead, that in the name of wellness, well-being and health, we have been fed incomplete information.

As an autoimmune warrior, I have walked the path.

I was a senior financial services professional, globetrotting, exceeding expectations and deadlines, winning awards and achieving success. I had a happy family life, a loving husband and a wonderful daughter. So why did I collapse one day and suddenly find myself with rheumatoid arthritis? My mother said I had a gene and my doctor said he couldn't pinpoint the reason as autoimmune conditions affect one per cent of the population (now, the number is much more). *But my mind was telling me it was stress.*

I was caught in the middle of a bubble of negativity. Apart from my family, the folks around me, whether at work or on the party circuit, were full of this negative energy. And like a sponge, I began absorbing it. It didn't affect the others, because just like we all look different, our responses to stress and disease are also different. So, one person may perceive a situation as perfectly normal while another is devastated by it. And that's what happened to me. The predictability of my life, body, mind and ability to function or enjoy life suddenly collapsed. I was in my weight range, I ate my vegetables, fruits, and exercised. I was what you would tout as 'healthy'. What was I doing wrong? The fact was that I did not sleep much and my response to stress was poor, and I had become a sponge absorbing negativity.

I was also an introvert pretending to be an extrovert.

I did not take charge of my stress till the crisis hit me, and when it hit me, it destroyed my quality of life. There are things I cannot do any longer which many healthy people, even older than I, are able to. I used to paint and hold exhibitions, but because of my damaged wrists, I lack the painstaking stamina it takes to create the details that bring alive a canvas. My brain fog has lifted, but parts of my brain have been engraved with the screams of pain I felt every single day. It was an irreversible change and I had to build my new life around what I *could* do. But what healed me wasn't just nutrition.

It was a shift in my own energy.

So, the first thing we need to do is step back and change the way we look at disease.

The number of people who fall ill and die in their 50s is increasing drastically every day. Look at these truths:

- Between 1990 and 2017, 5.15 million people died of cardiovascular disease between the ages of 50 and 69. And 3.96 million died of cancer[1].
- As per a joint report by the World Health Organization (WHO) and the World Economic Forum, lifestyle diseases account for almost sixty per cent of deaths worldwide and are responsible for almost forty-four per cent of premature deaths.
- Dyslipidaemia (abnormal levels of lipids like high triglycerides, high cholesterol) is one of the top contributors for lifestyle diseases and gets priority in funding studies.
- The number of adults with raised blood pressure increased from 594 million in 1975 to 1.13 billion in 2015, with the increase largely in low- and middle-income developing countries like India. With raised or fluctuating hypertension comes damage to the kidneys which often goes unnoticed until it is too late. In fact, information on the link between fluctuating hypertension and kidney damage is still low and sporadic.
- The role of raised or fluctuating blood pressure, as well as strange lesions on the kidneys for those who have been on inhibitors, has been a cause of concern for most hypertension patients in clinical data.

- Something as simple as a zinc deficiency has also been linked to being a trigger for hypertension[2]. This tiny, water-soluble nutrient that protects the immune system, when missing, can cause havoc that can so easily be prevented.
- With the presence of the risk factors for heart disease—hypertension, high lipids—comes the risk for type 2 diabetes, another deadly lifestyle disease.
- The number of people with type 2 diabetes globally is 422 million, as per WHO, and the global deaths associated with this disease is 1.6 million.
- Type 2 diabetes does not come in isolation—it is a major cause of blindness, kidney failure, heart attacks, stroke and lower limb amputation. In the 1970s, this disease used to be called late-stage-onset diabetes because it was a degenerative disease, affecting an older population. However, today it has morphed into a lifestyle disease. (Ironically, a healthy diet, regular physical activity, maintaining a normal body weight and avoiding tobacco use are very simple ways to prevent or delay the onset of type 2 diabetes.)

Whatever I have stated above is not completely unknown to you. And yet, how do we view good health?

We view good health as an absence of disease.

I know many 'healthy individuals' who say they are feeling fine and never bother to get a preventive health check-up done because they don't feel the 'need'. They also abuse their body and mind with these five excesses:

- Smoking
- Excess alcohol
- Excess food
- Excess stress
- Less sleep and rest

Yes, excess food is as much a malady as the rest. Combine that with the sedentary lifestyle that people have been moving to since the 1970s and the result is a burgeoning population of people under severe stress because of their work or relationships, who are at increased risk for lifestyle diseases.

How often have you heard of someone suddenly dying and people saying, 'He/she was fine, perfectly healthy.' They were 'healthy' because they didn't know about the triggers present inside them or they did not listen to their mind and body to see the signs before it was too late. I can recall many instances, the most prominent one being of the CEO of a global technology firm, bless his soul. He was within body weight range, ate healthy and exercised regularly, was lean and looked boyishly youthful, and yet, he collapsed from a sudden heart attack and died at just 42. He had also been an avid marathon runner. He seemed to be doing all the right things, but he wasn't getting any sleep. He slept for only four hours a day which means that two crucial criteria were missing in his life—sleep to repair him and reduced stress levels. He left behind his wife and small kids. During an interview with a business TV channel, just two months prior to his death, he was shown jogging and talking about the three pillars for 'physical well-being'.

As a holistic nutrition expert, I recognized that it wasn't just lack of sleep that was the problem but also this focus only on 'physical well-being.' We are not merely physical bodies but rather the amalgamation of our body, mind and soul. The moment you start understanding the interconnectivity between the three, the focus shifts to feeding each one. Skimping on rest and sleep is a sign that you are not nurturing yourself. This lack of respect for oneself is the common thread between people who fail to recognize the signs their mind and body are sending them. This tendency is especially seen in people who work too hard and are constantly striving to surpass themselves[3].

What used to be known as 'the highest earning years'—I would narrow this period down to between the ages of 50 and 60—has now become 'the most dangerous age'. Why is that? It is because in this stage of our lives, the pressure on people is the highest:

1. The kids are in school/college so there is financial pressure to pay fees or help them settle down.
2. You are at the top of your career. The demands of your work are at the highest because you're responsible for others or a business P&L (profit & loss).
3. You are the spouse of a stressed-out professional. As the spouse, you are absorbing the pressure and anxiety they feel, and anxiety for your future is even higher because you want to see your kids settled.
4. Your parents are growing old. Most of us are close to our parents and anyone with parents around 75 years of age or older, ends up having at least two incidents a year

of health crises pertaining to them to manage, whether you live with parents or are thousands of miles away.

5. You want to give your work that one last push. This is always the most damaging factor. You want to retire, and you keep telling yourself that you will practice some self-nurturing habits after you retire. Right now, your focus is to save up for a rosy retirement, which frankly may not fructify because you need to make it there alive. Apologies for the fatalism, but that, my friend, is the truth.

And it is not just this age group. As per a study by Vanderbilt University[4], indicators of despair—depression, suicidal ideation, drug use and alcohol abuse—are rising among those in their late 30s and early 40s, across most demographic groups. These findings suggest an increase in 'deaths of despair' in the youngest members of Generation X, that is, those who were born between the late 1960s and early 1980s.

When we are in the best state of health—physically and mentally aligned and balanced—our brain and organs secrete chemicals like dopamine, serotonin, endorphins, etc., that give us everyday joy. The brain is calmer, response to stress starts reducing and we don't get irritated or snap. The disease activity (reversible manifestations of the disease) inside becomes drastically lower, as evident in lower inflammation markers. We are less susceptible to colds, coughs, the flus, have a healthier beating heart, lower sugar levels, higher agility and mental sharpness and better moods. I'm not talking about achieving nirvana or becoming a sadhu; I am talking about reaching a state of equilibrium that will give you joy daily. And to reach there, let's examine your life.

If you are anywhere between the ages of 35 and 55, this could be your current life:

You wake up in the morning, trudge to the bathroom, get ready, gobble down breakfast, get to work, email, meetings, phone, then eat, more meetings, email, commute, phone, come home, eat, phone, sleep.

Repeat. Till Saturday morning.

And then suddenly on Saturday, you're catching up on your sleep deficit, still doing some work (even if it's just being on 'calls' as many would dismiss them to be), having one meal or doing some activity with the family and considering that as 'quality time'. And finally, there's the social weekend obligation to relatives or unwinding by enjoying food and drinks with friends before you hit the bed on Sunday night, as tired as you were on Saturday morning, as tired as you will be when you wake up on Monday morning.

You are working, earning a wonderful salary, have a good boss/business, a sound mind, and a supportive family. So, there is no problem.

Or is there?

Hey, what happened to rest, repair, rejuvenation, 'me-time'? What happened to pausing for yourself and letting your mind and body absorb a slower pace that will repair the damage of the week? How will you repair the damage? Why does it need to be repaired?

Because it is this kind of lifestyle which causes accelerated ageing. But we don't have the time to recognize the signs, we don't *want to* make the time. The only way we pause is if there is a calamity: we fall ill or a family member does, we get laid off, or there is a global pandemic that gives us enough time for reflection.

Why do human beings behave reactively rather than proactively? We were not born like this. Remember your childhood? You went out and played because you just enjoyed doing it and not because it was 'good for you' or something that mom told you to do. You played in the mud, climbed trees, even ate a little bit of the mud (without worrying about germs!), rolled on the floor with the dog for no reason except for the joy of the activity, and you cherished the happiness that these moments gave you. And then came the conditioning: don't do this; you'll get dirty. Don't climb trees; you'll get hurt. Go do your homework if you want to get good grades and get that game you've been asking for. The conditioning became a bribing system which started remapping a pure mind to a 'give-and-take' and reactive mode. Growing up, we're told that if we do something, we'll be rewarded with something better; if we work hard, we'll be successful.

Unfortunately, it is the same approach towards our health. If we fall ill, we go to the doctor. The doctor could be a medical doctor, Ayurveda specialist, homeopath, or the neighbourhood/family Mr/Mrs Agony Aunt. Whoever you went to, you were only taken to them when there was a 'problem'. So, you grew up thinking that you only need external help when there is a problem. You could solve all your problems on your own, failing which, one reached out, not before. For many of us, that means we drive ourselves to continuously seeking solutions even if we may be inept at finding them, and by the time we have reached a state of complete exhaustion because of our inability to find the solution, the damage has already been done. So, what are we missing in this entire conditioning?

We missed out on the journey. The joy in the every day. As children, we enjoyed the process and journey of getting dirty; that was what our 'driver' was. Our focus was not on having a bath afterwards. But today, when we look at our rewired brains, it is always the end which is the focus and not the journey. Whether you are working for somebody else, yourself or are unemployed, there is always an end picture which is rosy, perfect, like the California sunset, that propels you to put in your best, ignore your health and your sleep, because you've been conditioned to believe in that rosy picture, which is a mirage. And in that process, you're missing out on what you are creating every day, every moment of your life.

There is the compromised immune system threatened by a pandemic, the accelerated ageing that causes early disease, unexplained pains, chronic fatigue, brain fog, memory loss, bad skin, creaky joints … The list is endless. So, in this hurry to reach the rosy end, our present day, *this day*, and our daily activities become a chore. The *joie de vivre* every single day is missing.

Always remember, the end is not picture-perfect, the end picture is death. Or a life that leads to death. The only certainty in life is that we will all die. And as a human race, we are doing well in driving ourselves to that end faster than ever.

But we are alive today.

And life comes with an unpredictable, exciting promise. Every single day you wake up is an opportunity to create another beautiful day. Is it difficult? Of course, it is. Anything that pushes you out of your comfort zone—your brain is going to resist it. But the wonderful thing about our brain is the function of neuroplasticity. The brain adapts; it is the mind that tells the brain to adapt.

And the mind, my friend, is in *your* control.

So why is it difficult? It's difficult because again, we have been conditioned to look at our health as absence of disease. Till we are not hit by a health crisis, there is no such thing as, 'I will nurture myself and look after my mind and body daily to prevent disease.' Look around you, look at me. We are all creatures who have suffered and then adapted a path of preventive or curative healing.

Together, we can change this truth.

2

The Approach of Treatment

Ranjit Das, or Ronnie to family and friends, spent his 75th year running between different hospitals to find out what was ailing him. He had lung oedema, a condition in which the lungs fill up with water. Doctors would drain out his lungs, and he was given steroids, but the water would fill up again. He was admitted and tested at Fortis, AIIMs, National Institute of Tuberculosis and Respiratory Diseases, Apollo, and Sir Ganga Ram Hospital. There was no clear diagnosis, tests did not show it, but the fluid kept coming back, so doctors summarized it was cancer. All kinds of tests were done, from nuclear MRI, lymph node biopsies, blood work to check cancer markers and other scans. Finally, the Sir Ganga Ram Hospital oncology department, after extensive testing, ruled out cancer.

Ronnie was discharged after a year of tests, hospital bills and no clear diagnosis.

He decided that it was time for him to connect the dots himself. This was not the quality of life he wanted. He had always lived life on his own terms, right from his National Defence Academy days (he was preparing to become a naval officer but due to an unfortunate eye accident had to leave) to his work in the tea gardens, and then finally with Gillanders for thirty-eight years. Even after that, he worked with the Rajiv Gandhi Foundation first and then with the Family Planning Association of India, an NGO. He had always been the charming bachelor in high demand, was used to living by a schedule and a structure. Being left in the lurch at this age, without a diagnosis, was like an open-ended part of his life he was uncomfortable with.

So, he spoke to a few people. A medical worker who was a neighbour, some friends who were part of meditation groups, a few family members. He absorbed all the information. And then he came up with his own schedule:

- Ronnie had always been an early riser, so he wakes up at 5.30 a.m., does some freehand exercises, and twenty minutes of deep breathing in his garden.
- After that, he enjoys a cup of herbal tea.
- Then he cooks a lavish breakfast of porridge and seasonal fruits, along with either leftover kheema from last night's dinner, eggs and toast, or upma, as per his mood or availability.
- From 11 a.m. till 1 p.m. he cleans the entire house (he is extremely house-proud), including dusting, mopping, and making his bed. He doesn't have any household help.
- Lunch is usually very light as he is a small eater. Some rice and dal or sometimes nothing at all. Post-lunch is usually spent catching up with friends and loved ones. In pre-COVID-19 times, he would do that by driving

out, but now he uses Zoom. Conversations with nieces and nephews. And finally, in the evening, he attacks his kitchen with a passion to make some scrumptious dinner for himself, which he barely pecks on.

- A small dinner—tiny portions of a couple of spoons of rice, a couple of spoons of dal, two-three bites of some animal protein, and vegetables—only these chosen ones: cauliflower, cabbage, French beans, or carrots. Dinner is over by 8.30 p.m.
- At 9.30 p.m., he unwinds by pouring himself a small whisky. Has some more conversations or listens to music or watches the news. He enjoys his two 30 ml drinks over about an hour and a half.

At 81, Ronnie has no health issues. The lung oedema disappeared. Once a year, he gets a preventive health check-up done and takes vitamin D, B12, magnesium and selenium on a regular basis. He laughs when you talk to him about that one year of frantic doctor visits and lab tests. 'I needed to get to the bottom of this and that is why I went through with it instead of giving up. If it had been cancer, I would have dealt with it and got treatment. But I needed to know what it was.'

The fact that a Type A personality like Ronnie is happily content with living under the lockdown situation is perhaps the biggest testament to how far he has progressed on his health journey. His mind is not agitated by the restrictions; it is working its way around, making the best of his situation.

I asked him what was his biggest joy at this stage after conquering something that doctors could not diagnose. He says, 'Hang on!' and takes his phone (we were on a video call) to his terrace garden and shows off his peace lilies. 'It is 46°C over here, but look at these beautiful flowers,' he says proudly. 'I love spending time here, and now that I have got used to this quarantine schedule, it's a holiday—I may never go back to my old life.'

While Ronnie never got to know the cause of his ailment, he found the solution himself. He eats meat, enjoys his drink, has a few select vegetables and some fruits daily. He has the best doctors and hospitals at his disposal and yet he had nearly reached a dead end in his life. He is single. He defies everything you have ever heard of from a 'being healthy' perspective. He is not a vegetarian, drinks alcohol, lives alone—all of these are detrimental to health as per research.

And yet, he has not only fixed his health but is enjoying his daily life.

Ronnie has cut through the clutter of 'health gurus' and found his own path.

When I talked to Ronnie about younger people suffering from chronic health issues or suddenly dying, he said, 'These people gave up. They did not want to go to the root cause and get it fixed, they did not see the signs. When I had my problem, I wanted to get to the bottom of it. I was proactive.' Ronnie's journey showcases what we already know: there is a flaw in the way we look at our health. He did not find his answers with doctors, so took charge and is now living a flourishing life.

We keep running from diet to diet, one healing methodology to the next, or doctor to doctor. Fads are followed like religion. Whichever treatment methodology we turn to, ultimately our mindset is that of 'treatment', and not 'way of life'. This myopic view is costing us our quality of life and lives.

SCHOOLS OF HEALING

The role of various types of medicines or healing methodologies is different:

Western medicine

This is emergency medicine and is a reactive science. It can save lives because it was invented and created in times when, during the early twentieth century, we were losing populations of people to epidemics and pandemics. Hence, the methodology of treatment has been rooted in emergencies, natural disasters, plagues, flus, virus attacks, an unfortunate accident, getting physically hurt, and needing repair at a physical level.

The father of medicine, Hippocrates, was a medical practitioner from the Greek island of Kos, who lived in the fourth and fifth centuries BC. He became famous for developing the concept of humoral theory to explain why people became ill[5].

As per his theory, a healthy body has a balance of four 'humours' or fluids—black bile, yellow bile, blood and phlegm. This was the accepted explanation for disease triggers followed by doctors in Europe until the seventeenth century, over 2,000 years after Hippocrates.

Modern medicine, or medicine as we know it, started to emerge after the Industrial Revolution in the eighteenth century. At this time, there was rapid growth in economic activity in western Europe and the Americas.

During the nineteenth century, economic and industrial growth continued to develop, and mankind made many scientific discoveries and inventions[6]. Scientists made rapid progress in identifying and preventing illnesses and in understanding how bacteria and viruses work. And so, the primary purpose of modern or Western medicine was to treat infections.

Infectious diseases, viruses and bacteria led to the development of vaccinations. Then came World War I. Again, emergencies to save lives became the focus of modern medicine. Development of the first antibiotic, the first dialysis and the first chemotherapy drug took place in the 1940s, showcasing yet again that the focus of modern medicine was at the diagnosis stage. There was no preventive health research or focus except with 'alternative' healers.

And hence the principles of treatment were the same you would use to fix a machine, a broken-down car or torn blanket. Fix it if it breaks, repair it, and work towards getting better at fixing and repairing it when the damage has occurred. The energy, research and focus has always gone into how to fix it better at a physical level.

High cholesterol? Prescribe statins. Heart blockages? Remove them surgically through stents or a bypass surgery. Kidney damage due to type 2 diabetes? Kidney management medications, dialysis and finally a transplant. No health experts focus on the reversal process; they all talk about management with medication and half-hearted lifestyle changes.

The focal point then is, if there is a surgery, how can doctors be more precise with the surgical procedure with fastest rate of recovery? If there is a transplant, how can an organ from one body fit into another body with the least amount of resistance at the physical level? If there is a broken leg, how can we fix it to be almost back to its original form? If there is a virus, how can we find an antidote to ensure that the virus gets killed inside? These were and are pertinent areas of research and development for all medical researchers and scientists. They get the maximum research funding from pharmaceutical companies because the results will make a business case for higher sales. The role of going inwards, and naturally reactivating the ability of the human body to repair itself using nourishment in various forms, was always and continues to be missing.

Due to this, treatments were confined to the physical level, except recently when medical scientists acknowledged the role of the mind in patient recovery. So many people have been disillusioned with doctors without understanding the role of Western medicine in saving our lives. It is a self-limiting science dealing with physical repair work. Having expectations of a quality of life from an emergency treatment is a false expectation.

And yet, ironically, the father of Indian medicine, Hippocrates, is known for this quote: *'Let food be thy medicine and medicine be thy food.'*

Maybe he knew about Ayurveda?

Ayurveda

Ayurveda is an ancient science put down by the old sages for treatment of various ailments.

The difference between Western medicine and Ayurveda is in the approach and methodology itself. Ayurveda can be used as a reactive or preventive tool whereas modern medications and methodology can only be used as a reactive tool.

Since Ayurveda experts understood the medicinal properties of herbs and their healing impact on the human mind and body, they used purer forms of plant-based medicine with lower side effects. Toxicity of Ayurvedic medicine occurred when our soil became toxic or due to tampering by companies trying to sell substandard Ayurveda products. Thus, in some parts of the US, certain Ayurveda herbs were banned because of the presence of heavy metals, which are naturally present in the soil and have increased due to the pollutants in the soil.

Anyone who has read the basic principles of Ayurveda will agree that it understands the human body as holistic. And that differentiates Ayurveda from modern medicine. Today, when we are grappling with all kinds of diseases and many unknown ailments, the role of the gut in repairing the immune system is becoming important. We need to relearn from the ancient texts that Ayurvedic experts used, to bring back the health of the person by focusing on repairing the gut.

The fact that Ayurveda is seen as an alternative and complementary medicine field is ironical because even Western medicine experts are now turning to repairing the gut to reduce inflammation and increase immunity to treat most diseases. Many medicines made by Western medicine practitioners and pharmaceutical companies also come from plants and chemicals but are extracted and combined in a manner that increases potential side effects. But pharma companies or doctors are not even apologetic about it; they just print literature and expect the layperson to understand side effects and interactions that are based on too many variables like gender, age, other medications, emotional state of mind, etc. Basically, the risk is for the individual and the profits are for the pharma companies.

Homeopathy

Homeopathy was founded by Samuel Hahnemann (1755–1843), who studied medicine in Erlangen, Germany, in 1779, and died a millionaire in Paris in 1843[7]. He experimented with and came to the conclusion that if a patient had an illness, it could be cured by giving a medicine which, if given to a healthy person, would produce similar symptoms of that same illness but to a milder degree. For example, if someone was suffering from severe nausea, he was given a medicine which in a healthy person provoked mild nausea. This led to his famous aphorism, 'like cures like', and that became the genesis of homeopathy.

Like Ayurveda, the treatment methodology of homeopathy also focuses on plants, herbs, and minerals. It works on the premise that the human body can repair itself and activates repair mechanisms that stimulate the healing process. This system of treatment originated 200 years ago in Germany and is hence almost as new as Western medicine, possibly without the toxic side effects. I have seen homeopathy work wonderfully on children because their immune systems are not yet developed and can be manoeuvred to respond better to healing.

But, again, like Western medicine, and Ayurveda, our response to homeopathy is also reactive. If there is a problem, turn to homeopathy for a solution. Even though both Ayurveda and homeopathy can be practised for preventive health, very few people utilize this.

So, what is a reactive response? For example, when somebody pinches you, you react both at the physical level of pain and an emotional level of emitting negative energy towards the person who has pinched you. Similarly, we have a reactive response inbuilt to our body's signs. Unless there is a stimulus, we believe that status quo is good for us. But the human mind and body is not dormant. It is reacting to your thoughts, food, and conversations at different levels; there is the conscious or the gross mind and the subconscious or the subtle mind.

The gross mind sends signals for physical needs like hunger, cold, heat, desires, sleep, and physical discomfort. It governs at the physical level of the body, from birth to life to death and decay. The subtle mind, on the other hand, operates on energy. There is energy inside us which comes into existence much before the physical or gross body does. The entire universe functions on this energy and that is why it is an intelligent universe. People who operate at the gross mind and body level, operate with a reactive mode. Those who've managed to tap into their vital force, or subtle energy, run on a preventive and nurturing mode.

In my experience, I have seen both Ayurveda and homeopathy work with or without the support of Western medicine in a reactive manner. Which means that when there is a health crisis, one of these fields of treatment is applied with positive results. The other forms of complementary medicines like acupuncture, pranic healing, yoga and Reiki are supportive but also significant in their function.

One of the most remarkable things that has happened is the fact that what is often described as alternative, complementary medicine or sometimes quackery, has survived for centuries in a very wide variety of forms. This is because many practitioners and patients have seen the results for themselves in the healing process without side effects.

Today, the boundaries of complementary and modern medicine are blurring to respond to the demands of a sick world. Many medical doctors are turning to what is known as 'integrative medicine'. Integrative medicine neither rejects conventional medicine nor accepts alternative therapies uncritically.

The philosophy of integrative medicine[8] is:

- The patient and healer are partners in healing.
- Multiple things influence health—body, mind, spirit, and community.
- Use of both modern and alternative methods to heal.
- Natural, less-invasive interventions should be the priority.
- Along with treatment, prevention of illnesses is important.

Medicines, doctors, and hospitals are for emergency needs. The purpose of our life should be to prevent, manage and reverse health issues, and avoid medical emergencies and chronic lifestyle conditions. How?

Via holistic nutrition.

Integrative medicine is a holistic medical discipline that takes into account the lifestyle habits of the patient. The difference between holistic nutrition and integrative medicine is very little. Integrative medicine is treatment based on holistic nutrition and medicines to manage conditions. But holistic nutrition can prevent you from becoming a patient or help you recover completely, reducing dependency on drugs. In both scenarios, whether you are a patient or do not want to be one, holistic nutrition has the power to heal you.

Holistic nutritionists like me have long believed what doctors today finally concede—that modern medicine alone is not enough to alleviate disease or give back quality of life. We do not look at the human body, mind, and soul as separate because every aspect of our thought process, our actions, and what we put into our mind and body, impacts how we absorb nutrition. A holistic approach also considers your environment, your relationship with yourself and those around you, and your anxiety levels. This form of healing combines the power of Ayurveda herbs with natural, plant-based nutrients, the curative powers of yoga and breath work, and helps people create lasting habits. These blended lifestyle habits support the human mind and body in the process of repair and healing that changes gene expression. Yes, even if you have a genetic predisposition, holistic nutrition can change your gene expression to eliminate disease clinically from inside you via epigenetic changes, triggering repair.

Epigenetic healing repairs like the disease never existed.

The impact of holistic nutrition comes under the purview of epigenetics. This means that you may have genes to give you a particular disease or those that can predict whether you will have chronic health issues[9]. Holistic nutrition, however, modifies the response of your genes to prevent your risk of certain diseases or heal you in case you have already been diagnosed, like me.

I have seen cases where people with a specific cancer gene have been able to avoid the disease with their lifestyle changes, or somebody like me who had an autoimmune gene but was able to change the expression of my genes and not only overcome my incurable disease but also ensure much higher quality of life than Western medicine was offering me.

THE TWO PILLARS OF HOLISTIC NUTRITION

Physical nutrition

This is what you put inside your body in terms of food/toxins/pollutants/nutrients. Everything around us in the physical space is getting absorbed inside our body and mind. I meet many people who tell me that they eat organic or only apply natural, toxin-free products; they don't realize that they are still ingesting toxins. At a physical level, these toxins are coming from the air we breathe, the water we bathe with, the non-stick utensils we use; these are all absorbed by our gut and our largest organ—our skin. Releasing these toxins and eating nutrients that can reverse effects of toxins and disease is the purpose of each component of a holistic nutritional diet.

Just like the field of holistic nutrition, holistic treatment also has an integrated approach that factors food and the environment around us. The belief is—your relationship with food is as important as what you eat and how you eat it. Relationship with food is established as we grow up, and an unhealthy relation can lead to eating disorders like bulimia, anorexia, poor body image, etc. For instance, someone may have unhappy memories of eating with the family. Fixing this relationship aids better absorption, repair of the gut and immune system, and emotional conflicts.

Food can heal or trigger disease. The right blend of what you ingest to release toxins is imperative for the miracle of healing to begin.

Emotional nutrition

Our mind and thoughts make us who we are. Some factors that impact how you react or respond to stress, the health of your relationships, inflammation levels, and hormone levels, are:

1. Brain nutrients. These are naturally abundant in some and need to be added for others. These can reduce agitation and calm you down without use of drugs.
2. Childhood exposure to conflicts. This can influence your mind to make or break a relationship subconsciously. The relationship can be with yourself, your environment, food, or people.
3. Childhood exposure to perceived or real rejection— school jibes, bullying, or failure.
4. Your relationships with your parents, siblings, and self.
5. Your circle of friends growing up and what the dynamics were.

The field of holistic nutrition is vast and endless because the impact is so huge. In today's times, when we are grappling with our immune systems and avoiding a virus, disease or cancer, the role of holistic nutrition in strengthening our immune system and response to stress becomes even more pertinent.

Stress suppresses the immune system, and holistic nutrition impacts our emotions. Hence, the most obvious outcome of somebody who is holistically nourished is a high immunity and happiness quotient. And that is why, through this book, you will discover the delicate balance that can be attained with just *very simple habits* to find the joy in everyday living and leave disease activity, stress, anxiety, and conflicts far behind.

3

The Cost of Accelerated Ageing

In a world driven by economics, the cost of accelerated ageing is hitting societies that pay for healthcare much more than countries like India where the blow is taken by those who cannot afford insurance. That is sixty-six per cent of the population[10].

The top diseases that suck up medical expenses globally and in India are cardiovascular disease, type 2 diabetes, and cancer. Sadly, the first two are completely preventable, manageable, and reversible. And the last, cancer, is increasingly being linked to lifestyle factors, many of which are in our control. So, we can reduce the risk or accelerate recovery by adapting to a lifestyle that prepares us versus giving us a disease.

In September 2018, I was invited to London for a medical conference to deliver a talk on 'How to reduce the burden of diseases on hospitals and doctors'. I had been asked to share my case studies on preventing emergencies in type 2 diabetes and cardiovascular disease patients. These special case studies showcased how disease activity reduced clinically with better reports, lower inflammation, and lower markers like HbA1c, LDL cholesterol, and hypertension. Doctors globally are focusing on management of these better so that the patient is not rushed to the emergency room, as they are already overcrowded.

Today, as we face the pandemic, people with lifestyle diseases are more prone to catching the virus than people who are healthy. As per WHO, evidence till date suggests that two groups of people are at a higher risk of getting severe COVID-19 disease[11]. These are people over age 60 and those with underlying medical conditions like cardiovascular disease, diabetes, chronic respiratory disease, and cancer. WHO has issued advice for them for community support to ensure they are protected from COVID-19 without being isolated, stigmatized, left in a position of increased vulnerability or unable to access basic provisions and social care.

With 65 million people in India—and 9.3 per cent of the entire global population—being diabetic, the burden of care for type 2 diabetes is huge. Not just in managing sugar levels, but also damage to the kidneys (many diabetics require kidney transplants). If you combine that with the fact that the presence of type 2 diabetes as a risk factor for cardiovascular disease and vice versa, the common population at risk for any kind of collapse medically is very huge. As per WHO, 'Many people in low- and middle-income countries are detected late in the course of the disease and die younger from CVDs [cardiovascular disease] and other noncommunicable diseases, often in their most productive years'[12].

And the cost is not monetary alone. The trauma that the human body and mind go through in every episode of emergency, and the stress and anxiety caused to loved ones, are some of the costs we never account for. Rather than enjoying time with our loved ones and being healthy enough to work daily, our focus ends up on managing our health conditions. And that can lead to two things:

1. If you are a working professional, your capacity to work is going to start diminishing, making your organization wonder if they can get a younger, more agile version of you at a lower cost and replace you.
2. Sudden death.

With these two scenarios as inevitable, understanding how to make changes to avoid both is the path that any sensible person will take.

As per many published clinical research studies, people with type 2 diabetes can reverse the condition by following a low-calorie diet[13]. I have had cases where, in just a matter of four months, the HbA1c came down from 11 to 5.5. Below are a few facts to help you understand how type 2 diabetes manifests in the body:

1. Higher calorie intake or storage (due to long hours without food, skipping meals, overeating, a sedentary lifestyle) leads to excess fat in the liver.
2. Owing to this, the liver responds poorly to insulin and produces too much glucose.

3. Excessive fat in the liver is passed to the pancreas, causing insulin-producing cells to fail.
4. Losing just less than one gram of fat from the pancreas through diet can restart the normal production of insulin, hence reversing type 2 diabetes.

Imagine leaving behind the life of the diabetic—sluggish, at risk, worried about getting cuts and wounds, cardiovascular disease—and starting to live a life without worry? And a worry-free life is a happy life!

Cardiovascular disease experts like American cardiologist and researcher Dean Ornish have shown that heart disease is completely reversible without medication, with lifestyle corrections. A study, led by Ornish, demonstrated clearly that intensive lifestyle changes lead to regression of coronary atherosclerosis after one year[14]. Just one year. So instead of living with statins, beta-blockers, being worried about chest pain and keeping Sorbitrate at hand, it is easier to just get rid of this stress by making the disease disappear. This also cuts out the risk of type 2 diabetes and sudden death via a stroke.

Now let's look at cancer. Lifestyle behaviours and environmental factors account for around seventy to ninety per cent of cancer cases, according to research published in the journal *Nature* in December 2015[15]. The research concluded that only ten to thirty per cent of cancers were a result of a natural mutation. The rest—up to ninety per cent—were caused by external factors such as smoking, environmental toxins or dietary choices.

Research shows a link between development of cancers and our lifestyle/environment. In my last book, *You Can Beat Cancer*[16], I have shared my own case studies that reveal how a healthy diet can help in recovery of cancer survivors and improve their quality of life[17]. Patients came to me in both scenarios—those who did not want to get into conventional Western treatments and those who were undergoing conventional Western treatments. In both scenarios, not only was healing much faster, but we reduced chances of recurrence.

We achieved this by using integrative medicine[18]. While medicines prescribed by doctors were consumed, we focused on holistic nutrition to repair and reduce the side effects of medicines. It was only when the repair was demonstrated, both in symptomatic relief and blood reports and scans, that the doctors tapered off medicines systematically.

If somebody already damaged and ravaged by cancer can respond to this kind of treatment so well, imagine how a healthy human mind and body that wants to prevent cancer will respond.

So, what is the mantra to prevent or reverse health conditions? Is it a one-size-fits-all?

In an earlier chapter, we met Ronnie, who took charge of his health following a lung oedema. Ronnie is doing everything wrong as per health gurus touting pillars of longevity and good health. These are listed below:

1. Ronnie doesn't eat too many vegetables. Most health experts talk about eating five portions of vegetables.
2. Ronnie eats meat. Most diets, fads, health gurus promote veganism.

3. Ronnie is single. Most studies show that loneliness can cause diseases, even kill. But he overcame his.
4. Ronnie drinks whisky. Every day.

And yet, Ronnie overcame what doctors couldn't treat. By changing his focus and energy. With the power of his mind.

Part 2

The Mind

Making up your mind to do something
is the most powerful tool towards
a healthier life.

1

Your Mind is Your Immune System

Laurence Nossein is 53 years old and lives in the suburbs of Paris. For twenty-five years, she was on antidepressants. After being diagnosed for anxiety following a dizzy spell, the doctor gave her a low dosage and asked her to continue taking it.

Laurence did not have a good marriage but could not walk out because she had two young daughters and her husband was suffering from multiple sclerosis. But as years went by, she began to feel more stifled by the toxicity of the relationship. When her daughters were 16 and 18 respectively, Laurence finally decided to leave her husband. What drove her to seek a divorce was concern for her own health. 'My health in the relationship was suffering and my husband's health has been deteriorating because of his condition. I was not happy in the relationship but had stayed on because I felt guilty about leaving a sick man,' Laurence confessed. 'But the fear of our daughters not having even one parent to fall back on in case they underwent some kind of a crisis, finally made me gather the strength to take this decision,' she admits, adding, 'for the first two months I cried every day. I felt I had split the family, destroyed it. I was very guilty. Six months later it became better. I don't regret it.'

But something miraculous happened after Laurence was done with the crying. She quit taking the antidepressants and never felt the need to go back to them. Twenty-five years of dependency vanished in a moment.

The mind has strange ways of helping us cope. In a toxic relationship, some of us need the support of drugs, food, alcohol, or other substances to deal with the emotional toxicity. The toxicity could be in a personal relationship, at our workplace or even with our own business. Sometimes, many are unaware of this toxicity but are absorbing it at a subconscious level.

But when we free ourselves from this negativity, the mind adapts, becomes stronger and helps us live a more fulfilling life. When that acceptance happens, we break away, like Laurence did. Today, she is content mentally. In her soul. She's serene and focusing on her emotional health. Earlier, the thought of ageing scared her. 'A lot of things we don't need, let us not accumulate,' she says, in her charming French-laced English. 'I am going to shift from Paris to a house in the mountains with trees, because I love trees. God has been kind: I have never had painful periods, I had a very easy birth with both my daughters, very swift, and I recovered very fast,' she says. Ask her about her food and she eats healthy, except when it comes to dessert.

'I don't like fruit as dessert; I want real dessert, sometimes chocolate spread,' she says, 'I am French, after all.' Red wine with friends is twice a month. Her boyfriend is with her on the weekend. 'We walk every weekend, hiking in the woods, 15-20 km, and I do yoga twice a week. Recently I began jumping rope to get a three-minute cardio workout in twice a week.'

Till now, everyone has told you that if you eat right you will not get diseases. If you protect your immune system, you will be able to avoid or overcome COVID-19 better. If you strengthen your immune system, you can avoid cancer or overcome it faster.

The role of the immune system is linked to everything we do and yet, treatment is piecemeal. Have this symptom, take this tablet. Let us take a step back to understand what we mean when we say, 'Strengthen your immune system'. Every day your immune system destroys a cell that would have become cancerous if it lived. The five things that influence this process are: what your skin absorbs, what you ingest, how you breathe, how much you move and most of all—*what you think*.

THE POWER OF CHOOSING YOUR THOUGHTS

Nurturing the immune system means making your mind stronger with both physical and emotional inputs. Consider the following scenarios:

1. Somebody who eats right has been shown to succumb to diseases.
2. People who exercise regularly are getting diseases.
3. People who meditate but don't eat right are prone to getting diseases.
4. People who eat home-cooked food frequently get lifestyle diseases.

5. People who eat right, meditate and exercise regularly but live in fear, get diseases and infections.

Of course, there are benefits of eating healthy, exercising right, and doing your meditation, but what is the balance that can change your response to stress and strengthen your immune system?

The balance is in your emotional state.

This balance is not the obsession with doing things right; the balance is the attitude of incorporating practices in your lifestyle, as habits, without letting them consume you. The most important thing all the people that I have talked to have in common is their attitude. And it is this attitude, this shedding of fear, that has helped people reach a positive outcome and enjoy every moment without finding any of these activities to be a chore. *They are in harmony with themselves.* Lack of harmony is what triggers a conflict in our minds, leading to emotional response or reactions.

So how do we get in sync with our emotions? And why is it important?

Emotions can be negative or positive

In any given situation, different people react or respond differently. Consider the following scenario:

There is a traffic jam and two senior business leaders, Ajit and Vipin, are stuck in traffic. Both are getting late for a very important meeting. Ajit gets agitated. He is, after all, a leader who must set an example for his team by being punctual. He starts pushing the driver to take shortcuts but there is no way out. All through the nearly one hour he is stuck in the jam, his anxiety is rising. He is sending frantic messages to his team. He asks them to be on standby because he is trying his best to make it to office. Even as Ajit urges the driver to cut through, deep down he knows he can do nothing about it. His frustration is building. This frustration gets transferred to the driver and in his nervousness, the driver bangs the vehicle in front of him. This causes the owner of the vehicle in front to come out and start fighting with the driver and Ajit. A traffic cop comes over to help. The driver of the other vehicle wants to take Ajit and his driver to the police station. After twenty minutes of heated discussion, the matter is resolved. But this altercation has only caused Ajit further delay.

Sitting in the same traffic jam, Vipin, on the other hand, starts chatting with his driver. After assessing that there is no way out, Vipin decides to put on his headphones to catch up on the classical jazz he enjoys but never really gets time to listen to, and he opens his laptop to respond to pending emails. Like Ajit, he also sends a message to his team. 'It seems like I'm going to be on the road for a while, why don't you guys have a cup of coffee or tea and grab a bite because we are going to start a little late.' His team members are thrilled, there is a relaxed atmosphere and people catch up on their emails while enjoying their coffee. The hurried pace has slowed down a bit, allowing everyone time to have a calmer morning.

When both reach their offices, the atmosphere in the two meetings is diametrically opposite. Vipin's team is relaxed and able to come up with creative ideas and is receptive to his presentation. The meeting ends quite quickly because everybody is working as a team *in harmony* and because there is positivity in the room, and delegation of tasks is faster and amiable. Ajit, however, reaches office in the same agitated state and finds a bunch of wary colleagues. He is not able to communicate the wonderful initiatives in his presentation because he is not relaxed. In short, the task at hand faces a small setback and more time is spent convincing his teammates to get on board.

As somebody who has worked in the corporate sector in a senior position and now works with senior business leaders helping them with their health, I can share that the above scenarios are, unfortunately, real. There are very few organizations that understand and percolate down the importance of reducing stress levels to increase productivity. Apart from reduction in productivity, health of the employees is at risk.

Experiencing frustration, anxiety, fear, and stress is considered a normal part of life when it is occasional and temporary, such as feeling anxious and stressed before an exam or a job interview. However, when those acute emotional reactions become more frequent or chronic, they can significantly interfere with daily living activities such as work, school, and relationships. Chronic stress is a pathological state that is caused by a prolonged acute stress response and can wreak havoc on our immune, metabolic, and cardiovascular systems, and lead to degeneration of the brain's hippocampus[19].

Worse still, anxiety immediately leads to overproduction of acids in the stomach, compromising digestion. If the cycle of anxiety is not broken, continuous overproduction of acids leads to killing of good bacteria, high acidity, bloating, lower absorption of nutrients from food, constipation and finally, a compromised immune system. Many of the senior executives whom I have treated are unaware of the overproduction of these acids. The focus for most organizations, and hence employees, is to finish more tasks in less time, which in itself will compromise output. Pushing an anxious employee to multitask a compromised output of productivity is detrimental to the employee because it reflects in his or her review assessments. It also impacts the organization—when a company is being run by emotionally agitated employees, you can expect poor decision-making. Interventions like exercise, mindfulness training, and cognitive behavioural therapy reduce this pathological anxiety and stress and decrease risk of developing disorders.

In fact, science supports the theory of an unhurried pace in comparison to multitasking.

'Not only do people experience stress with multitasking, but their faces may also express unpleasant emotions and that can have negative consequences for the entire office culture,' said Ioannis Pavlidis, director of the Computational Physiology Laboratory at the University of Houston, and senior author of a study[20] conducted in May 2020 about the emotional impact of multitasking in a work-from-home environment during the COVID-19 pandemic.

It's common for office workers to juggle multiple tasks at once. But those constant interruptions can create sadness and fear and, eventually, a tense working environment. This does not mean that multitasking is bad or shouldn't be done—the brain and neurons can be trained to perform such tasks without agitation, with higher effectiveness. But experiencing unpleasant or negative emotions has an adverse impact on relationships, whether at work, home or within oneself.

Negative emotions feed negativity

We have all heard about positive and negative emotions. But what do these emotions do for us? If I am reacting negatively to the environment or people around me, I will emit negative energy. Which is what Ajit did. But if I am in harmony with who I am inside myself, my external environment and people's negativity will not impact me. I will emit positive energy. And this is what Vipin did.

Quantum physics says the entire universe is an intelligent universe made up of these energies. We are part of a vast, invisible field of energy that responds to our thoughts and feelings. Think about it—every physical thing in our life is not just solid matter but rather, fields of energy or frequency patterns of information. Every human being, along with every material thing in the universe, broadcasts a distinct energy pattern, and this energy carries information. In short, we are all interconnected[21]. Every human being emits a specific energy pattern. Our fluctuating mind, conscious or subconscious, changes this pattern on a second-to-second basis because we are not just a physical body; we are consciousness using a body and a brain to express different levels of the mind.

It is a well-known fact in various civilizations and cultures that all our planet's oceans are connected. In one of my chats with Dr Alejandro Junger, a functional medicine doctor and cardiologist based in Los Angeles, he shared a conversation he'd had with a native American spiritual leader. 'If I touch the water in my city, the water in Los Angeles is connected to the water in the Arabian Sea where you are, in spirit,' he said, sharing that the ancient cultures believe in this and so does he. Dr Junger instituted the Clean Program where the focus is on cleaning your gut to repair your health.

If what quantum physics and ancient cultures say is true, there is also *proof* of this in recent effects of energy healing with chronic diseases patients. Researchers have found strong evidence that biofield therapies like Reiki reduce pain intensity and are effective at lowering pain in hospitalized patients as well as in patients with cancer[22]. There is evidence that these therapies ease agitated behaviours in dementia and anxiety in hospitalized patients.

What Laurence experienced was negative energy from her spouse which created toxicity and need for antidepressants. But the positive energy from her children gave her the strength to walk out and live her life. Energy, then, is both a function of what you absorb and how your mind reacts to it. The moment the negative energy vanished from Laurence's life, so did her dependency on antidepressants.

There have been so many documented cases of caregivers or family members going into depression or contracting serious illnesses themselves after the person they were caring for passed away. They absorbed the negativity, experienced compassion fatigue and this manifested physically in the form of illness. Diseases have a physical manifestation but the genesis is in the mind, something that's been proven by researchers at the University of Virginia School of Medicine, who determined that the brain is directly connected to the immune system by vessels previously thought not to exist[23].

The mind can assess if an emotion is negative or positive. But there is a physical impact of feeling these emotions on our physical body. Imagine this scenario: you are on a new date or in a large client meeting. You experience butterflies in your stomach, which is a real and physical impact of an emotional response. The fear of disease, viral infections, loss of a loved one, fear of being judged, all create physical impact by giving us anything from palpitations to dry mouth to sweating to a sinking feeling in the chest or stomach. Similarly, positive emotions also have an impact: imagine a gooey, dark chocolate cake or ice cream waiting for you in the refrigerator. Your emotional response of craving it creates saliva in your mouth. Hence, it is wrong to say that what we feel does not affect us physically. Our thought processes have already shown they affect us physically by secreting hormones, triggering bodily functions like a bad stomach or frequent urination when, for example, one runs away from a barking dog out of fear. These are all physical reactions and not recognizing that emotions drive our physical state is the biggest folly we make when we look at our well-being.

If for such momentary things, the physical reaction can be so evident, imagine the response of our body to chronic stress. A bad relationship for years, a job that does not appreciate you, a business that no longer excites you. *All these create a feeling of lack of self-worth and make you neglect yourself.* Self-nurturing habits like me time, exercising, deep breathing and nourishing yourself all take a back seat and overeating, or starving, substance abuse in the form of food, alcohol or smoking become common patterns. There are physical ramifications of negative emotions which, when combined with lack of healthy living, finally trigger disease.

Everything is controlled by the mind

The mind is the centre of our being. Our ability to fight disease, find a solution to a twisted problem, overcome physical health issues, endure pain, reduce stress and anxiety so that we can live a better quality of life, are all governed by the mind. The mind is not an organ—no doctor can pinpoint where the mind is located. It is not the brain; the mind controls the brain. Physical manifestations of an agitated and stressed-out brain, like hypertension, clinical depression and aggressive behaviour have been recorded; mind–body interventions like yoga and meditation help in reducing these manifestations, symptoms and help repair at the DNA level. In fact, mind–body interventions (MBIs) don't simply relax us, they can 'reverse' the molecular reactions in our DNA which cause ill-health and depression, as per studies[24].

Millions of people around the world already believe in and practice the health benefits of MBIs like yoga, pranayama or meditation, but what they don't realize is that these benefits begin at a molecular level and can change the way our genetic code responds. It is a wonderful way of helping your mind change gene expressions and control disease response.

Living a life without agitation can alter the immune system

When you are strengthening your immune system, the inputs you are providing will pacify your brain and reduce anxiety levels so that you can aid the process of clearer thinking without agitation. This life without agitation is an altered response to stress—stress itself never goes away—but we can change our response to stress to repair the immune system by reducing anxiety, strengthening the gut, and making absorption of nutrients higher. A stronger mind, then, means a stronger gut and higher nutrient status in the blood, leading to a clinically stronger immune system and reduced inflammation.

People who experience anxiety benefit by regulating microorganisms in their gut by consuming probiotic foods and supplements, which reduces their anxiety[25]. We have trillions of microorganisms in the gut which perform important functions in the immune system and aid metabolism by providing essential inflammatory mediators, nutrients and vitamins—these can help regulate brain function through something called the 'gut–brain axis'.

And that gut–brain connect is controlled by the mind because the mind can reduce anxiety and inflammation. The biggest function of the mind is to reduce inflammation, which is the most potent cause of diseases, low quality of life and early death. Remap your mind and you can control inflammation levels, and an inflammatory response. Across all fields of treatment—medical science, clinical research, nutritional science, Ayurveda, homeopathy, MBIs—the common consensus is about inflammation being the root cause of disease and poor quality of life. Anxiety, stress, fear, poor sleep, poor nutrient status, and lack of activity, all contribute to this inflammation.

2

Stress and Our Mind

Stress always manifests in the human body as a symptom, an effect. These symptoms can be controlled when we control stress levels. Symptoms of chronic stress are inflammation that triggers diseases, which leads to poor quality of life, depression, and finally the lack of will to live. This lack of will is the final push towards death from a life that could have been lived well.

CONTROLLING THE CAUSES CONTROLS THE SYMPTOMS

Stress changes the structure of the brain. During a stressful event, the stress hormone norepinephrine suppresses a molecular pathway that normally produces a protein, GluA1, without which nerve cells and astrocytes cannot communicate with each other[26]. This communication breakdown creates disharmony in the mind, triggering stress-induced changes which include accelerated ageing and increased inflammation in the brain and other body parts, leading to parameters for depression and lifestyle diseases to rise. In people who are already immunosuppressed or compromised, the trigger of stress is enough to cause a flare-up, increased pain levels, recurrence of cancer, brain haemorrhage, sudden heart attack or a stroke.

And stress is contagious.

As if we did not have a contagious virus and pandemic to deal with, it turns out even stress can be transmitted from me to you under certain circumstances[27]. If you are living with a stressed-out partner, for example, that stress is likely getting transferred to you. So, in a way it's everybody's responsibility to reduce stress levels for the entire family. How many times have you heard of people in the same family falling ill in quick succession? There is growing evidence that caregivers of patients with cardiovascular disease are vulnerable to developing their own poor cardiovascular health, investigators report in the *Canadian Journal of Cardiology*. This is due to compassion fatigue, and it is common even in therapists and practitioners like me, where we experience extreme fatigue after absorbing the negativity or stress of our patients.

'Compassion fatigue is a state experienced by those helping people or animals in distress; it is an extreme state of tension and preoccupation with the suffering of those being helped to the degree that it can create a secondary traumatic stress for the helper,' says Dr Charles Figley, professor and director at the US-based Tulane University Traumatology Institute.

Many relationships and families reach a breakdown stage because of the state of chronic stress of one individual passing it to the entire family. It can result in separations, divorces, children being brought up in a state of constant stress because of the lack of a nurturing environment, who in turn grow up to have high risk of lifestyle diseases and depression.

Symptoms of compassion fatigue include[28]:

Work related

1. Avoidance or dread of working with certain colleagues/clients/tasks given
2. Reduced inability to feel empathy towards people
3. Frequent use of sick days
4. Lack of joyfulness

Physical

1. Headaches
2. Digestive problems—diarrhoea, constipation, upset stomach
3. Muscle tension
4. Sleep disturbances—inability to sleep, insomnia, too much sleep
5. Fatigue
6. Cardiac symptoms—chest pain/pressure, palpitations, and tachycardia

Emotional

1. Mood swings
2. Restlessness
3. Irritability
4. Oversensitivity
5. Anxiety
6. Excessive use of substances: nicotine, alcohol, illicit/self-prescription drugs
7. Depression

8. Anger and resentment
9. Loss of objectivity
10. Memory issues
11. Poor concentration, focus, and judgement

If you are experiencing any of these symptoms, this is what you need to do to start cleansing yourself.

1. **Self-care first** Nourishment provides emotional stability. Breathing techniques can be especially helpful to cleanse yourself of negative emotional energy that causes compassion fatigue. 'Caring for someone with a chronic ailment or disability requires physical, mental and emotional commitment by the caregiver. It takes your time, energy and effort, which is an exhausting investment and causes fatigue,' says Dr Bhavana Gautam, a mental well-being specialist from Mumbai. She helps caregivers establish self-care boundaries and runs her own online sessions on anxiety release.

2. **Set emotional boundaries** This is extremely important. This means structuring your day to include me time. Carve out some time every single day to be on your own to stay grounded within.

3. **Engage in outside hobbies** All work and no play makes Jack a dull boy, so only working and thinking about work is going to make you feel pessimistic and lower your energy. Find something other than work that you enjoy; practice that and practice self-nurturing.

4. **Cultivate healthy friendships outside of work** You need to have a perspective of the outside world,

even outside of your immediate family. This not only refreshes the mind and body but also gives you fresh perspectives on other people, helping you grow as an individual. Friendships, physical or virtual, can be sustained with constant communication and time spent with each other. In today's world of video calls and Zoom parties, this is increasingly possible!

5. **Keep a journal** If you are feeling overwhelmed, putting something down on paper always helps get all the negative energy out and makes you feel lighter. Keeping a journal has been clinically shown to reduce anxiety.

6. **Use positive coping strategies** These include pranayama, meditation, and gentle exercise. Apart from nourishing yourself with healthy food and lots of vegetables, start practising gentle yoga and you will realize your response to stress begins changing. And once that happens, you become calmer at work and home, making everyone seek you out for advice/work/fun time.

If not reversed, compassion fatigue can lead to depression. And depression is the disease of the twenty-first century, as evidenced by WHO and depression-related suicides that are on the rise.

Depression is real

Depression is a common mental disorder affecting more than 264 million people worldwide. It is characterized by persistent sadness and a lack of interest or pleasure in previously rewarding or enjoyable activities. It can also disturb sleep and appetite; tiredness and poor concentration are common in depressed people. The causes of depression include complex interactions between social, psychological, and biological factors. Life events, such as childhood adversity, losing a loved one or unemployment contribute to and can trigger the development of depression. Close to eight lakh people die due to suicide every year, which is one person every forty seconds. There are indications that for each adult who died by suicide, there may have been more than twenty others who attempted suicide. In 2016, seventy-nine per cent of suicides occurred in low- and middle-income countries. Suicide accounted for 1.4 per cent of all deaths worldwide, making it the eighteenth leading cause of death in 2016.

Psychological and pharmacological treatments exist for moderate and severe depression. However, in low- and middle-income countries, treatment and support services for depression are often absent or underdeveloped. An estimated 76–85 per cent of people suffering from mental disorders in these countries lack access to the treatment they need[29].

And what can help with depression? A breathing-based meditation practice known as Sudarshan Kriya Yoga helped alleviate severe depression in people who did not fully respond to antidepressant treatments as per a study[30].

Poor sleep is a big risk factor for triggering depression. So how does sleep affect our mind?

3

Sleep and the Mind

William Shakespeare was not just a brilliant writer; he had a profound understanding of the human psyche that influenced the detailing of each character in his plays. His work transcends time and is relatable even today because he understood the psychology of the human mind.

Shakespeare's biggest contribution, as far as I'm concerned, is his description of sleep (in *Macbeth*) as the 'balm of hurt minds'. We carry our hurt and grudges inside us which lead to a building up of anxiety and stress. Sleep helps us absorb and gain a perspective on whatever may be bothering us—a person, situation, or comment. We have been told so many times, 'Sleep over it.' It is the best advice anybody can give to reduce response to stress.

There is another rhythm, apart from the circadian rhythm, which rewires the brain.

The circadian rhythm is the naturally built-in twenty-four-hour clock that times our biological rhythms, including sleep cycles. Scientists have found the part in the brain where this rhythm is generated. But there are two systems regulating sleep in the mind—one is the circadian rhythm and the other is the homoeostatic system.

The homoeostatic system induces and pushes us to sleep depending upon the intensity of activity our brains have undertaken. If the brain is working overtime to maintain equilibrium when it is over wired, you suddenly find yourself exhausted and fall asleep for a few hours from sheer mental exhaustion. This is because your brain has been in a chronic state of stress and is exhausted. This exhaustion is different from the exhaustion that comes from physical work or learning, which makes you feel satisfied and gratified, resulting in sleep that is sounder and for a longer period. That kind of sleep rewires and rejuvenates the brain. However, sleep for the constantly worrying brain comes in spurts and is disturbed sleep, which is why we end up waking tired, because the rejuvenation has not happened.

SLEEP CONTROLS BRAIN AGEING

Before physical, accelerated ageing takes place, there is mental or brain ageing which can trigger the physical ageing process. Ageing is controlled by the hypothalamus, which regulates our hormones and metabolism. Due to age, disease, stress, and lack of sleep, neural cells in the hypothalamus that control ageing begin to die. And when that happens, the brain starts getting into a stage of accelerated ageing. Not surprisingly then, researchers at Duke-NUS Graduate Medical School, Singapore, found evidence that the less old adults sleep, the faster their brains age[31]. These findings, relevant in the context of the world's rapidly ageing population, show the path for loss of sleep and its effect on memory decline, dementia, and Alzheimer's.

Less sleep has been found to affect the heart, raise sugar levels, and make a person enter a prediabetic stage, increase cravings for sweet food, which further feeds accelerated ageing. Just ensuring seven to eight hours of sound sleep is a wonderful preventive solution to reducing brain ageing and risk for diseases. This is corroborated by the fact that inflammatory changes in the hypothalamus can increase risk of metabolic syndrome—a syndrome wherein a combination of health problems can lead to heart disease and diabetes[32].

Dr Lydia DonCarlos, a neuroendocrinologist and professor at the Department of Cell and Molecular Physiology at Loyola University Chicago's Stritch School of Medicine, studied how hormones affect the structure of the brain. Hormone production by the hypothalamus needs to be efficient as hormones govern body temperature, hunger, stress responses, sex drive, circadian rhythms, and sleep. DonCarlos and her colleagues examined data from 320 studies reporting sleep duration findings for healthy individuals, effects of reduced or prolonged sleep duration, and health consequences of too much or too little sleep. And after finding the impact on the human body, the expert panel recommended that teens (ages 14 to 17) get eight to ten hours of sleep per night and adults sleep for seven to nine hours[33].

Do you know anyone who sleeps for eight hours every day, consistently?

Problems like mood swings, acne, hormonal issues, and depression in teenagers are on the rise. The correlation between brain agitation and lack of sleep makes it clear that just getting the right amount of sleep can start reversing these problems; and we can have a generation of healthier teenagers, and correspondingly, a generation of healthier parents with lower response to stress. A large part of the stress of parents is due to the health problems of their children. Ironically, the more successful people get, the less soundly they sleep. In the case of women, less sleep triggers hormonal fluctuations leading to hormonal issues and an increased risk of hormonal cancers[34], and depression. Fortunately, neural cells can be rejuvenated and the process of the neural cells getting affected by lack of sleep is reversible.

SLEEP AND DISEASES: A FEW FACTS

- **Insufficient sleep amplifies levels of anxiety** And, conversely, deep sleep helps reduce such stress[35]. A full night of good sleep stabilizes emotions, whereas a sleepless night can trigger up to a thirty per cent rise in anxiety levels, according to research from the University of California, Berkeley. Deep sleep seems to be a natural *anxiety inhibitor*, so long as we get it every night consistently. For people who can't get good sleep, doing MBIs like gentle yoga and breath work, provides calm and consistent sleep over time. Yet, these are almost never recommended to those who seek help for anxiety and stress.

- **We have an entire generation of teenagers and millennials brought up on low sleep** Anxiety is common in teenagers and youngsters, but a good night's sleep has been shown to reduce that response to stress, as per a Michigan State University study. This is the first study to identify that sleep helps adolescents cope with stress.

- **Lack of sleep causes hormonal distress** Today, hormonal disruptions and depression in the young is robbing them of their quality of life. Lack of sleep alters hormones, metabolism—which governs the rate of burning calories—and triggers accelerated ageing in young people. Chronic sleep loss can reduce the capacity for basic metabolic functions such as processing and storing carbohydrates or regulating hormone secretion in adults as well[36]. This means that the body can go into fat storage and create fluctuating hormones that can lead to hormonal disorders like malfunction of the thyroid and polycystic ovary syndrome (PCOS). It's been a very long time since I met a woman who did not have either of these issues. In men, it can lead to reduced sex drive, lowered self-confidence, and obesity. And obesity is a risk factor for heart disease and cancer as clinically proven. The good news? The moment people with hormonal disruptions go back to a consistent good night's sleep, they start reversing the process of these disruptions and conditions in just four days. We are already dealing with endocrine disruptors; we need the support of good sleep to be able to flush them out and give the body a chance to repair and rejuvenate itself.

- **Sleep loss increases cravings** People who sleep less than four hours a day have suppressed leptin levels, a hormone that regulates appetite[37]. As hunger levels due to lack of sleep increase, food choices change. After two nights of curtailed sleep, a study found volunteers craving candy, cookies, and cake. Lower levels of sleep increase appetite and cravings, leading to that midnight sweet snack—and obesity. With these erratic habits comes hormonal fluctuation which can alter a person's mood and rob them of the opportunity to live a better quality of life. This should be a wake-up call for parents. In the strive for perfection for their children to get higher marks or excel at multiple activities at the same time, the compromise of sleep is going to cost the child heavily throughout their lives.

- **Less sleep can trigger heart issues** For stressed-out working professionals, less sleep in middle-age triggers hypertension, stroke, and sudden heart attacks. It is sad that organizations are not putting pressure on employees to sleep a minimum of eight hours a day because if they do that, productivity of employees will be higher and number of working hours will be less leading to lower insurance costs. Lack of sleep means poor health, costly diseases, emergencies, and hospitals.

The good news? These are all *reversible* when we consistently follow the plan to sleep well.

How to ensure you get a good night's sleep

Most of us struggle either with going to sleep or getting up within a few hours and not being able to go back to sleep. Whichever one you are struggling with, listed ahead are some of the tricks and techniques to help you sleep better.

Get your magnesium levels checked Very often, magnesium deficiency causes insomnia and cramps. A simple blood test can check your levels and you can take prescription magnesium supplements. If you are deficit, you will need 500 mg magnesium before sleeping every night. Most women will also benefit from this supplementation in reducing menstrual cramps and hormonal fluctuations. Foods naturally rich in magnesium include raw almonds, flaxseed, tofu, chickpeas, dark chocolate, and avocados.

Stop caffeine at 5 p.m. If you are a coffee or tea addict, caffeine can interfere with sleep if taken after five in the evening. All cola drinks and energy drinks also have high quantities of caffeine. Ideally, you should not consume carbonated drinks at all, as they can strip your gut and increase risk of pancreatic cancer. Regarding coffee and tea, limit these to two in a day and do not take them after 5 p.m.

Eat early One of the biggest reasons for disturbed sleep is eating late. You may fall asleep immediately after dinner, but this sleep will be unfulfilling, and you will wake up tired. Eating by 7 p.m. and sleeping by 10 p.m. is ideal. Sleeping on a relatively empty stomach will mean that your digestive system is calm, which will aid deeper sleep.

Be rigid about your bedtime The simplest habit to make sure you feel sleepy at the same time, and can doze off without difficulty, is to set a bedtime. After a week to ten days of doing this, your body clock changes and you will start feeling sleepy at that time. Initially, when you get into bed, not being used to sleeping at that time, you will toss and turn. However, as days go by, this forced habit will start becoming a natural habit. Starting to sleep early is the first step towards rejuvenating and repairing damage to the body and heart and reducing stress levels.

Keep that phone away You would have read enough to know that the blue light emitted by cell phones disturbs our circadian rhythm; for stressed-out people, this couldn't be worse. Your phone should always be in another room. Initially, you will get separation anxiety; this is very common. It is a sign of addiction. For everyone addicted to their phone, keeping the phone on silent in another room will make them feel restless. It is fine; when you are changing a habit, a few days of discomfort for a lifetime of good health is worth it. After ten days of doing this, you will look forward to detaching from the phone and enjoying your me time in bed.

Bring some chamomile to bed Chamomile is a great gut pacifier and induces natural drowsiness. Add some organic honey which is full of natural probiotics and minerals, and your tummy will be so happy that it will send a message to the rest of your brain and body to doze off.

A happy tummy helps you sleep better Eating by 7 p.m. and having chamomile tea at 10 p.m. are both steps to ensure your food is digested by the time you sleep and your stomach and digestive system get a chance to rest. Our digestive system is our second brain. If we keep it happy, our sleep quality will improve drastically, leading to better repair and rejuvenation. Hence, the above habits will ensure that you have a happy tummy by the time you snooze off.

4

Fear and Your Mind

Dr Nandini Guha is a 65-year-old retired college professor. She came to me with severe pain and rheumatoid arthritis. She began improving within the first two weeks of treatment and then suddenly disappeared. Since that rarely happens with my patients, I got in touch with her son. He and I had a long conversation where he shared that his mom was continuously crying every few minutes throughout the day since the diagnosis of his father's Alzheimer's. I asked him to set up another session for her with me. So, a time was set.

From our earlier sessions, I remembered Dr Nandini as a well-composed, retired history teacher. This time, when she came on Zoom, she was nervous, her hands were shaking, and her palms were sweaty. I asked her what happened. It was like she had been waiting for me to ask, and she burst into tears. I let her cry for five minutes and then gently said, 'You have let it out, now you need to tell me what happened. You have to express it in words.' She had a few sips of water and whispered to me, 'My husband has been diagnosed with Alzheimer's. My son is a cancer survivor. He underwent a second scare.

And now I'm scared my husband will forget me and my son will die.' So deep-rooted was her fear that she was expressing herself as if these things were certain to happen.

I asked her to step back and think about what the senior college teacher Dr Nandini would have done if this were somebody else's family. What advice would she give a student, friend or relative in the same situation? Her teary eyes suddenly began to clear up and she started talking.

'I would have asked them to take charge and seek help to make sure that the health of their loved ones did not deteriorate,' she said. As she was saying this to me, her own realization hit her. I smiled, continued the conversation for another half an hour. I gave her five things to do for the next fifteen days to reduce her fear and distract her with physical activities. These activities also reduced inflammation, anxiety and pulse rate, and increased oxytocin and adrenaline, which helped calm her mind.

Fifteen days later, when I did another session with her, she said, 'I had lost my sense of reasoning and logic.' I did not agree, and gently told her that fear had overpowered her mind and had led to this situation. I had given her calming techniques, foods and exercises which worked together to reduce her fear and help her think calmly.

So, what advice did I give her?

To remap her mind.

A team of researchers under the guidance of the University of Bonn Hospital in Germany was able to demonstrate in a study that the bonding hormone oxytocin inhibits the fear centre in the brain and allows fear stimuli to subside more easily[38].

Oxytocin is a hormone produced by the hypothalamus and secreted by the pituitary gland. When a baby sucks at the mother's breast, oxytocin secretion causes the milk to release so the baby can feed. At the same time, oxytocin is released into the brain to stimulate further oxytocin production. It is a chemical messenger in the brain, controlling key aspects of the reproductive system, including childbirth and lactation, and aspects of human behaviour[39]. In the case of Nandini, who is 65, this natural production had reduced drastically, and the anxiety of her circumstances suppressed it further.

FEAR IS OF TWO KINDS: LEARNT AND INNATE

Innate fear is coded in our brains while learnt fear is what has impacted our memory via a traumatic experience. For example, if a dog bit a child, and the fear wasn't addressed in childhood by, say, adopting a dog as a pet, fear of dogs can continue during adulthood. Many years ago, I had a fear of cold, damp places because in my mind such places were associated with the extreme pain I experienced during my rheumatoid arthritis years. I had to consciously work on visiting places with cold and damp weather, like London, and creating happy memories in the same weather to overcome this fear.

Learnt fear can always be overcome with a systematic approach of the mind. With innate fear, however, it is more difficult. Fight or flight is an inbuilt response we are born with to immediate danger like a loud noise, falling, an object being hurled at, etc., that triggers an instinctive protective response. But fear of losing a loved one, spiders, cockroaches, of being unsuccessful, alone, in the dark, etc., are all learnt fears. Since we are all wired differently, some people make these learnt fears into an adventure and map their memory with reward. Extreme sports practitioners feel elated and release dopamine when they survive an extreme sport that most people would be terrified to try. Their reward is a sense of achievement and superiority over the larger risk-averse population.

Whether fear is innate or learnt, it produces anxiety. One of the primary reasons for anxiety disorders is the inability to overcome our fears for certain contexts in our lives that may no longer exist. While that has propelled the discovery of opioid compounds, which assist in masking fear memory, the mind is strong enough to be trained and change the context of the fear and overlay it with different memories[40]. The unfortunate effect of antidepressants is that in the first few weeks before the numbing sets in, the disorder is aggravated and hence, this treatment becomes counterproductive.

Anxiety fed by fear becomes chronic if neurons are not remapped.

Stress can be temporary but is a problem when it becomes chronic stress, also known as anxiety. A common form of anxiety, known as phobic anxiety, was associated with shorter telomeres (for more on telomeres, see p. 68) in middle-aged and older women. This means that if you are fearful as a person, you are going to age faster and will be at increased risk of lifestyle diseases. Just reducing this phobic anxiety will lower your chances of getting lifestyle diseases and cancer. Why should you need to have a deadly disease like cancer to start reducing anxiety? When we set our mind to change responses to stress, something incredible happens.

Our DNA begins to respond and repair.

5

Your Mind Can Repair Your DNA

When we are young and healthy, our telomeres are long. Epigenetic changes which include inputs from a good or bad lifestyle on the genes can alter the length of these telomeres. As telomeres shorten, risk of cancer and degenerative diseases increases. Evidence suggests that stabilizing telomeres slows down ageing and disease[41].

When inflammation starts increasing and risk of diseases shoots up, there are genetic changes that take place inside us. These changes can shorten the length of telomeres, which, like the tiny plastic tips on shoelaces, are protein complexes at the end of chromosomes. Shortened telomere length means accelerated ageing and risk of diseases. The inputs of sirtuin proteins, which are controlled by our anti-ageing gene, SIRT1, can regulate or reduce the ageing and disease process. And what impacts this?

MBIs like pranayama, meditation, and gentle yoga. Just like there are studies that show that the length of telomeres shortened due to stress (quoted in the previous chapter), there are studies that prove lengthening of telomeres after just three months of MBIs. Dr Linda E. Carlson, PhD, principal investigator and director of research in the Psychosocial Resources Department at the Tom Baker Cancer Centre, and researchers at the University of Calgary Department of Oncology, did a study on women with breast cancer[42]. And after just three months of MBIs, they saw the telomere length increasing. 'It was surprising that we could see any difference in telomere length at all over the three-month period studied. This is an exciting discovery,' said Dr Carlson. Eighty-eight breast cancer survivors who had completed their treatments for at least three months were involved for the duration of the study. The average age was 55 and most participants had ended treatment two years prior.

To be eligible, they also had to be experiencing significant levels of emotional distress.

There were two groups. In the mindfulness-based cancer recovery group, participants attended eight weekly, ninety-minute group sessions that provided instruction on mindfulness meditation and gentle Hatha Yoga, with the goal of cultivating non-judgemental awareness of the present moment. Participants were also asked to practise meditation and yoga at home for forty-five minutes daily.

In the Supportive Expressive Therapy group, participants met for ninety minutes weekly for twelve weeks and were encouraged to talk openly about their concerns and feelings. The objectives were to build mutual support and to guide women in expressing a wide range of both difficult and positive emotions, rather than suppressing or repressing them.

The participants randomly placed in the control group attended one six-hour stress management seminar. All study participants had their blood analysed and telomere length measured before and after the interventions.

Allison McPherson, one of the attendees of the group, was first diagnosed with breast cancer in 2008. When she joined the study, she was placed in the mindfulness-based cancer recovery group. Today, she says the experience was life-changing. 'I was sceptical and thought it was a bunch of hocus-pocus,' says McPherson, who underwent a full year of chemotherapy and numerous surgeries. 'But I now practice mindfulness and it's reminded me to become less reactive and kinder towards myself and others.' Study participant Deanne David was also placed in the mindfulness group. 'I think people involved in their own cancer journey would benefit from learning more about mindfulness and connecting with others who are going through the same things,' she says.

The key phrase here is 'become less reactive and kinder towards myself and others'. Just imagine a world where each one of us had lesser response to stress, which automatically increases our kindness quotient for ourselves and others. Wouldn't the world be a wonderful place to live in? And wouldn't we all sleep better, reduce our rate of diseases, and increase the joy in everyday living?

HERE'S HOW STRESS CAN SLOW DOWN YOUR AGEING

- A study published in *The Lancet* proved that changes in diet, exercise, stress management, and social support may result in longer telomeres[43]. These lifestyle changes included a plant-based diet (high in fruits, vegetables and unrefined grains, and low in fat and refined carbohydrates); moderate exercise (walking thirty minutes a day, six days a week); stress reduction (gentle yoga-based stretching, breathing, and meditation). So simple, right?

- Simple daily meditation can lead to improved cognitive functioning and lower levels of depression for caregivers.
- In a University of California study[44], it was clinically proven that daily meditation for twelve minutes a day for eight weeks increased telomere length, demonstrating slower cellular ageing. The results were 'striking', said Dr Helen Lavretsky, professor of psychiatry at UCLA's Semel Institute for Neuroscience and Human Behavior. Improvements were in mental health, cognition, and telomerase activity. The biggest improvement was seen with Kirtan Kriya that had several elements of using chanting, mudras (finger poses), and visualization. There was a 'brain fitness' effect in addition to stress-reduction.

Seeing this proof, you can now remap your mind to change your response to stress. Let's do it.

6

How to Make Your Mind Strong

Even if you are the most driven person on Earth your motivation can fizzle out depending upon your state of mind and body. But with discipline, the inclination to reach your goals becomes easier.

So how do you strengthen the mind if you don't know where to start? You can't immediately start meditating. You're setting yourself up for failure. You will do it for one week, maybe twenty days, and then give it up. Why? Because our mind is initially agitated and sitting in meditation requires calmness. This calmness is achieved by a structure because the mind and immune system always respond to a continuous structure. Children who are brought up in a structured environment have a stronger immunity and better response to stress.

If you have not been brought up to follow a structured routine or are not used to a structured day, it's never too late to begin. The mind adapts and *because* the mind adapts, the body adapts. The body does not exist in isolation—the directive is always controlled by the mind.

Cut the cycle of stress in the following ways:

DO BREATHING EXERCISES. DAILY

Pranayama is the method of extension and control of breath and helps bring conscious awareness to breathing patterns. This is part of MBIs and is the most powerful way to remap your brain and reduce its agitation. Once we have captured the fluctuations of the mind, the command over the body is easier. Breathing exercises have also been shown to reduce high blood pressure, high cholesterol, high sugar levels, depression, anxiety, stomach disorders (because it repairs the digestive system), and promote better sleep. With so many benefits, it is no wonder that all studies on MBI in chronic disease patients, including cancer, have helped with DNA repair.

For people who are already healthy, just regular deep breathing works. However, if you are stressed out and have not paid attention to your health, you need a structured programme for reducing mind fluctuations and inflammation levels. And while pranayama is good, all kinds of pranayama are not necessarily good for everyone. When we are stressed out and anxious, only cooling pranayama need to be done. These are: Anulom Vilom or Alternate Nose Breathing; Sheetali or Cooling Breath; and Bhramari or the Humming Bee breathing exercise (see p. 76-80).

Build an exercise plan

How you do these exercises, in what order, and for how long is the key. Like I said above, if you are in a perfect state of health and only need to do these from a maintenance perspective, you can do fifty counts and get the benefits of alternate nose breathing, and do five counts each of cooling breath and humming bee. However, in the following scenarios, you need to have a more structured schedule:

1. You have a lot of work stress.
2. You feel burdened with responsibilities.
3. You feel overwhelmed, irrespective of your age.
4. You have hormonal fluctuations evident in PCOS/ hypothyroidism mood swings, painful periods, hair fall, or acne (any one of these).
5. You have hypertension, type 2 diabetes, or high cholesterol already.
6. You get acidity or constipation a couple of times a month.
7. You wake up tired at least two days a week.
8. Often you don't know where the day has gone and there is so much left to do.
9. The lockdown has made you anxious and fearful.
10. You are a caregiver to older/ageing parents, a loved one.
11. You have teenaged children.
12. You are overweight.
13. Your sleep quality is poor, evident by daytime sleepiness or tiredness.
14. You feel fatigued often.
15. You experience brain fog.

If you experience even five out of these fifteen, the schedule below is going to help you get the energy, freshness, and quality of sleep to change your response to stress.

What you need to do to prepare

1. **You need quiet me time** This could be first thing in the morning, just before dinner, in the car when you are in traffic or, if you are lucky, sitting in an open place like your terrace, a park, a garden or by the beach. The last three scenarios are ideal, not mandatory. You need a clear twenty minutes. Without interruptions, calls, people coming in.

2. **You need music** Without music, your mind will initially wander. Choose music you love, it could be soft music of any kind—devotional, romantic, Sufi or some instrumental jazz. Whatever music you choose, make sure it is soothing and of slow tempo.

3. **You need a comfortable chair or bed** This is easily done whether you are at home/office/in the car. If you have access to a terrace, carry your cushion with you— the cold concrete can get uncomfortable and you don't want your mind wandering towards this discomfort. For people with back issues, you will need a chair or a sitting position that supports your back to avoid the distraction of back pain. Whichever way you sit, whether supported or without, please make sure that your spine is straight. The spine is the funnel through which the flow of energy takes place and the breath work will increase the flow of positive energy through this funnel.

4. **You need water** When you initially build up breathing exercises, your mouth is going to be dry and your brain is going to feel a little buzzed. This is because you are starting a new exercise. Remember when you start a

new fitness regimen? Your body reacts by resisting it, followed by stiffness and, later on, aches and pains. You brush it off saying this is muscle soreness associated with new exercise. It is the same with any brain exercises. Hence, keep a glass/bottle of water with you and when you feel dehydrated or dizzy, take one or two sips, not more.

Ready? Let us begin.

Sheetali or Cooling Breath

Sheetali has been clinically shown to reduce blood pressure in chronic hypertensive patients. Reducing high blood pressure is the first line of treatment to protect your organs and reduce inflammation levels. Sheetali cannot be done in cold climates outside or when you have cold, cough, fever, or flu. If you live in a cold country/city, and you are hypertensive, the ambient room temperature (in a heated room) should be 24°C. Do not step out into the cold immediately after doing this.

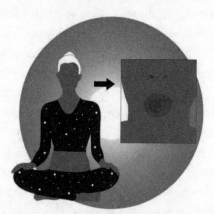

Do 10 rounds of Sheetali

1. Roll your tongue to form a tube.
2. Breathe slowly and deeply through the tube-like tongue.
3. Close your mouth at the end of inhalation and slowly exhale through your nose.
4. Repeat the same process for ten slow breaths daily.

Anulom Vilom or Alternate Nose Breathing

1. Sit in a comfortable position with your back straight and hands resting sideways on the knees. Even if you are supporting your back, your back should not be slouched, it should be straight.
2. Always begin from the left nostril. Close the right nostril with your right thumb and inhale slowly to fill up your lungs. The inhalation should not be forceful, it should be gentle but deep. Now, exhale slowly from the right nostril. Similarly, with exhalation, it should be gentle, unhurried, and flowing.
3. Inhale back from the right nostril in the same gentle manner, hold for two seconds and exhale deeply and evenly from the left nostril. If you are a heart patient, do not hold for two seconds; for everybody else, this is beneficial.
4. Inhale again from the left and hold for two seconds, and exhale from the right.
5. Repeat this cycle for five minutes, slowly, deeply, without hurrying. Remember: hurry is your enemy.
6. After five minutes, take a couple of sips of water.
7. For those whose arm gets tired, prop yourself with pillows to support the arms.

8. On the first day, only do five minutes. Build up two minutes every day until you get to fifteen minutes. And then do fifteen minutes every single day.

9. For people with chronic anxiety or depression, this should be repeated twice a day—once in the morning upon waking up and again at 5 p.m.

Regularly practised, these exercises have extraordinary health benefits in reducing anxiety and negativity. Within three weeks, you will begin to experience calmness and positivity and your pulse rate and blood pressure will drop. This reduces response to stress, inflammation, and repairs your gut.

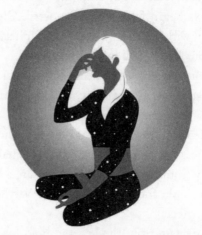

Do 15 minutes Anulom Vilom pranayama

Bhramari or Humming Bee

1. Close your mouth and keep the teeth slightly apart. Bring the tip of your tongue to the space behind the front teeth. Maintain this position of the mouth

throughout the practice, frequently checking to ensure that the jaw remains relaxed.

2. Close each ear with the thumbs, place the index fingers at the centre of the forehead—just above the eyebrows—and stretch the middle, ring, and pinkie fingers across the eyes so that the tips of these fingers press gently against the bridge of the nose.

3. Now, take a long, deep breath in through the nostrils, bringing the breath all the way into the belly.
   Begin to exhale slowly, making a steady, low-pitched 'Ommmmmmmm' sound at the back of the throat—like the humming of a bee. Focus on making the sound soft, smooth, and steady.

The positioning of the tongue encourages the vibration to resonate throughout your brain, cleansing and rejuvenating it. Keep your awareness on the centre of your head; you need to let the sound fill up your brain and feel the vibrations

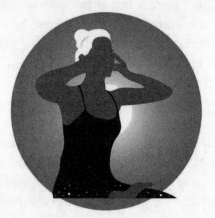

Do 10 rounds of Bhramari

on the sides of your face. Begin with five long repetitions. Slowly build this up to ten, and as you practise daily, you will realize that each repetition or exhalation of breath will become longer. Ideally, each repetition should be one-minute long and this can be achieved after a month of daily practise.

These three exercises need to be done in the order listed above. An ideal mix when you are building up these breathing techniques daily should be five minutes of cooling breath, fifteen minutes of alternate nose breathing and five minutes of humming bee. This is required to start reducing inflammation levels almost immediately along with repairing your gut. Consistency and regularity to get these results is a must.

CREATE A STRUCTURE

You can do your breathing exercises daily but that's just twenty-five minutes a day. Creating mindful habits throughout the day, on the other hand, is tougher but not impossible.

A day without proper structure is always going to cause anxiety because there is fear of the unknown. This fear may be in your subconscious and you may not be addressing it. Creating a fixed structure six days a week helps us break down tasks to a predictable daily flow. Once you create the structure, everything will seem like an errand to finish. And the moment your mind sees things as a task or errand, your brain takes over to finish these tasks. At that stage, the stress of the unknown, the anxiety of being judged, and negative emotions take a back seat. And you can focus positively on what you need to accomplish. This accomplishment will bring a sense of satisfaction which is very important to reduce stress and anxiety daily.

People who create and operate by a structure are often business leaders, visionaries, and coaches. In fact, research has proven that you can hack your brain to form good habits by simply repeating actions until they become a habit, according to a psychological research study from the University of Warwick.[25] Building a mathematical model of simple repetition can lead to good habits and an enhanced quality of life. Good habits like eating on time, sleeping on time, moderate exercise, and finishing your work on time lead to a balance between mind and body. Once this balance is created, and repeated daily, you can prevent, manage, and/or reverse any kind of disease.

On Sunday, your phone calendar should have the entire week mapped, with flexibility of two hours a day, a breather for emergencies.

Below is how you can create a structure in your life to reduce anxiety about the immediate future. I have used it to create health plans for senior leaders with amazing results, despite them being short on time.

1. **Set sequential tasks** This makes the day predictable, and helps your mind get more creative. Unpredictability compromises the mind and body because they will be in a state of conflict. Hence, creating sequential tasks is the first step towards conquering your mind to direct the body.

2. **Set eating times** Whether you are hungry or not, eating small quantities at a specific time will keep your metabolic rate high, sugar levels low, digestive system intact. This will also help you take a break. This is

important especially if you already have inflammation or any mild or chronic condition. Eat a small-portioned breakfast at 10 a.m.; a snack at 12.30 p.m., preferably something like fruit and ten pieces of almonds or pistachios with a cup of green tea; and lunch by 2 p.m., which should definitely include one vegetable, one salad/soup, a very small portion of your preferred carbohydrate, and a small portion of protein. If you have acidity, avoid wheat, lentils, and pulses, and go for vegetables, salad, and a small portion—five or six tablespoons, say—of boiled brown rice. Small portions will keep your digestive system efficient and your brain active.

Remember: more carbohydrates mean a sluggish brain. At teatime, 5 p.m., one cup green tea with fruit and nuts. Nuts are brain food, you must have them in between, but monitor quantities and do not soak them. Your brain needs the B vitamins which are destroyed by soaking the nuts. Dinner should be a small bowl/ cup of any vegetable soup, an even smaller portion of any preferred carbohydrate and protein. Remember: a small dinner will help you sleep better. Dinner should also definitely finish by 7 p.m. because you need to give your digestive system a break from 7 p.m. till 10 a.m. A minimum gap of fifteen hours between dinner and breakfast is essential to repair and rejuvenate the digestive system and expel toxins. This keeps the brain agile, and helps you sleep better.

STOP MULTITASKING

When we multitask, there are parallel tracks of information running in the brain; if the brain has a lower nutrient status or high stress levels, its ability to respond to each track efficiently is compromised. Hence, in initial stages of strengthening your mind and brain, you must start becoming more mindful of doing one task at a time. That activity will de-clutter your mind and make brain fog disappear. Please remember that brain fog is created in two scenarios—when our mind is fatigued or when we have chronic pain. In both scenarios, our mind is representing the immune system not running optimally. As someone who used to propagate multitasking and take pride in it, I changed my own habits long ago and revel in the here and now.

DISASSOCIATE FROM FEAR

Think of the worst-case scenario and internalize it. Then prepare yourself for it by saving up or stocking up (could be food/medicines/money, as per your fears). The worst won't come, but you're already prepared. If the fear is financial, sit down and look at the odds and plan your finances accordingly. For a temporary period, you can pare down your dreams of a lavish life or a bigger house and focus more on savings. In any case, we don't need most of the things that we acquire as material comforts. Learning to live with less will give you more happiness than you think. And making it into a happy path of living with less will also help you experience gratitude for all the blessings that you have already.

Play the deep breath game

You can institute time before dinner or breakfast and put on some music that everybody enjoys and start playing this game with everyone doing twenty deep breaths. The person who is the slowest, yes, the *slowest* and not the fastest, and finishes last, is the winner. This means they are taking long and deep breaths. Make sure there is a reward for the winner. The reward could be something small and not materialistic. It could be a special dessert for an older person; if it is a child, extra time reading stories in bed. Doing this will help your entire family reduce their response to stress. Over a period of time, everybody will be less stressed out. Playing games together will also strengthen your family bonds and affection.

Include de-stressing brain foods

Fresh green vegetables, whole organic eggs, extra virgin olive oil, flaxseed oil, avocados, oily fish, nuts, and seeds are brain-calming foods that reduce stress. Along with breathing exercises, if these foods are consumed, the brain gets nourishment to reduce stress.

Toss up a wonderful salad of freshly washed greens like salad leaves, lettuce, fresh chopped coriander/parsley/celery. Add flaxseed oil or extra virgin olive oil, a handful of crushed almonds and some chia seeds, crack some pepper, add sea salt. A large bowl of this kind of salad, every day at dinner, will go a long way in improving your family's overall health—especially for moody teenagers and ageing parents.

INCREASE BRAIN HYDRATION

Brain cells dehydrate faster than the rest of the body. Drinking one glass of water every ninety minutes of waking time is the best way to keep the brain calm and the circulation going. When the body's circulation is steady, blood pressure does not increase, and we stay cool. Whether it's adults or kids, inculcate this habit in every family member and put an alarm on your phone to observe water time!

DO MODERATE EXERCISE

The power of moderate exercise has never been explained fully. When we don't exercise or over-exercise, the body's response is inflammatory as there is oxidative stress. In contrast, moderate exercise calms the blood pressure; starts regenerating neurons, thereby improving memory and brain alertness; increases balance which in turn also impacts confidence levels; and is a mood lifter. With so many benefits, moderate exercise every day, along with the above habits, will ensure that your response to stress reduces.

So, what constitutes moderate exercise? An ideal combination is a moderately paced walk—not too fast, not too slow—every alternate day with gentle yoga. Follow this up with breathing exercises every single day. This balance is the MBI which can repair your DNA, reduce stress levels, strengthen the heart, and reduce inflammation. Whether you have a chronic health condition or not, this combination works for every person in healing themselves.

Remember, the mind's ability to heal the body is extremely high. All you need to do is follow simple and practical steps every day, day after day, to start feeling the repair work. Inconsistency in input is going to compromise the output, so don't cheat yourself. This is your time to heal yourself, and in doing that, a delightful thing will happen—your mood will be more positive. You will have higher energy, a verve for life, more empathy and gratitude, faster brainpower and finally, you will rediscover the joy of being alive.

This mind–body connection brings gratitude, an important aspect to live a fulfilling life.

Part 3

The Body

The body gets hurt even when there
is no physical harm.

1

Our Body Is a Subset of the Earth

We are constantly in a state of conflict, not just with ourselves but also with nature. We have overconsumed, overused, and abused our body just like we have the Earth.

Our health is linked to the health of the planet. The pandemic we are facing and how we emerge from it is going to have a lasting impact on how we treat the Earth. The moment we begin to respect nature, this intelligent universe we are in will give back to us. The more we continue to abuse the planet, animals, and other living beings, the more negatively it will impact the human race.

With so many people dying from the coronavirus, cardiac arrest, cancer, respiratory failure, depression, and other diseases, we have learnt that the impact of nature can be harsh and cruel. We need to go back to frugality, balance, and natural nourishment methods, and people like Ronnie, Steven, Laurence and many more that you will read about will teach us how we can. They are not wellness or meditation gurus.

How the mind–body are connected

To live this kind of life, the impact of stress on the human body needs to be understood. We must recognize that we are not merely a body; our thoughts too can trigger disease. Often, a physical symptom or disease is just a manifestation of what happens to us emotionally. Did you know there is something known as a broken heart syndrome?

Broken heart syndrome can occur from highly stressful events like the death of a loved one, a serious medical diagnosis, financial crisis, divorce, etc., discovered Loyola University Health System cardiologist Sara Sirna in 2015[45]. The medical name for this is stress-induced cardiomyopathy, Takosubo's cardiomyopathy or transient apical ballooning syndrome. The underlying cause is not known but is thought to be secondary to the release of excess adrenalin and other stress hormones that have a negative physical effect on the heart. Symptoms include chest pain, difficult breathing, and this can easily be mistaken for a heart attack. Broken heart syndrome typically occurs in patients older than 50 and is more common in women, although it also can occur in younger women and men.

So, what was initially thought to be a body with body parts that could be treated part by part, ended up having a trigger in the mind.

The good news is that this body can repair itself. The results of this repair can be proven clinically in the form of dissolved blockages, lowered inflammation markers, and in-range reports. A weak joint that may have been pronounced as needing replacement starts functioning well after holistic nutrition treatment; the muscles and nerves around the joint repair and support it to perform better and pain levels reduce. Some of my older patients who were advised joint replacement surgeries by doctors were able to reverse their diagnosis by following a holistic nutrition programme for six to eight months; they saw pain levels reduce and mobility increase.

And that is why you hear of people with physical debilitations who can push their bodies to perform tasks and activities thought to be impossible by medical science.

I have been through it myself.

Despite my 'teda meda' (twisted) bones and joints, I decided to do the gruelling 200-hour yoga teacher training certification. Of course, it was not without doubt, hesitation, anxiety, and fear.

As I strode confidently into The Yoga Institute, Santacruz East, Mumbai, on 1 November 2019, the serene environment and energy filled my heart with gratitude and positivity. All the voices from the last two months began to echo in my head as I approached my class.

Why are you doing this to yourself?

You can't bend much. Yoga teachers bend like rubber; you're stiff.

Do you like torturing yourself? (this from my mom)

You are a rheumatoid arthritis patient.

What about your deformities?

You must be realistic about what you can do and what you cannot.

You don't need to do this. You're healthy.

This is as good as you'll get.

The last thought rankled me. It was limiting me.

It continued for a few weeks through September and October while I was making up my mind and gathering my strength to take up the commitment for the yoga teacher training programme. I wanted to do it; nothing convinced me not to do it, but I was unsure of my body—could I rely on it? My mind was strong, but my body had a different view. I had been practising yoga for twelve years in my dilapidated manner to heal myself. It was the combination of nutrition, yoga and finally, my breath work, that pushed the disease activity outside my body. But not before leaving the scars of deformed toes, ankles, and damaged wrists. One of the orthopaedics we know saw my wrists' X-ray and laughed. 'If I didn't know it was yours, I would've thought *this patient* has no movement and no mobility and is in extreme pain. I would have thought *this patient* needs surgery,' he said. I also laughed and we both left it at that.

I could not sit in Vajrasana; my stiff spine needed support for Chakrasana; and I needed a modified cobra pose because my wrists couldn't take the load. A faulty Suryanamaskar schedule was done because my hands and wrists could not take my physical body weight in four out of the twelve poses to complete the process. In short, I could never be a yoga guru who has the poise, posture, and correct demonstration capability to bend like rubber. And yet I did yoga for twelve years and now I was going to expose myself to hundreds of people, admit to my compromised physical capabilities, and accept that I may not pass because I was not what you would expect a yoga teacher to be. With these uncertainties, I decided to go and have a conversation with the institute authorities.

The fear of failure loomed large.

I had to wait for a couple of hours like a good student to meet my course instructor, Manijaji. She had just too much work and too many students relying on her, loving her, and being greedy about their time with her. When I met her, I understood why. I went into a monologue about my deformities, my mother's health, my inability to do certain asanas ... After an exhausting one-sided conversation, Manijaji just looked at me, smiled, and said, 'This course is perfect for you.' The confidence of this young woman, who was fifteen years younger than me, gave me the confidence to push my body to the limit I was scared to push it to because of fear of failure. She kept brushing everything aside and saying, 'Just start and you will not only pass but also become a wonderful yoga teacher.' It gave me confidence. *She* had the confidence.

I tried again. My mother was undergoing health fluctuations and I knew I needed to be on standby if required. Manijaji told me that getting away for a couple of days because of a medical emergency would not be a problem. I spoke to my mom about it and she was very comfortable and reassured me that it was unlikely that during these 200 hours spread across thirty days, there would be any requirement for me to rush to her. Her positivity gave me confidence.

My friends and business partners had a mixed response. How long are you going to be away? How will you check your emails? There are patients who need you. Only one of them, Prachi, looked at me and smiled gently. 'You need to do this,' she said. 'Just do it.' She was not scared for me. She trusted the resilience within me. My husband Vikram was the other person who said, 'If you want to do it so badly, just get it out of your system. We will deal with it.' Years of living with me had taught him that my mind had been made up, and so I needed to do it.

So here I was, in my class, in my fiftieth year, as an autoimmune patient, with people half my age (or less), ready to start my yoga teacher training.

I was taught to work with my deformities rather than against them, with my body's consent rather than in discomfort, and I learnt about the mind–body connect even more deeply. The environment of the institute instilled serenity that started repairing me at levels I did not know needed repair. But ultimately, it was my decision to overcome my fear of failure that made me a certified yoga teacher.

It was the best decision of my life.

I learnt how to do thirty Suryanamaskars at one go without feeling pain in my wrists. I learnt how to do Utkatasana (something I could not do earlier), and stay in that asana, for a full two minutes. I was taught a simpler way to do Vajrasana by putting a cushion under my legs to protect my toes and I can sit in that asana now.

I can do the full cobra pose—my wrists support me!

I learnt specific asanas to open my spine and make it more flexible.

We were taught the principles of Ayurveda diet and that learning is propelling me to study Ayurveda and get certified.

The biggest learning I had was that to be a yoga teacher, you need to have the right knowledge of the mind–body connection. You do not need to bend like rubber to intimidate your students but gently help them understand this connection with the techniques taught in the course.

THE BODY REPAIRS, BUT THE KEY IS TO BE SEQUENTIAL

Have you ever cut your finger? Broken a bone? Has it ever happened that they have not healed? The body has an innate ability to heal itself. To heal a cut, we take precautions to not put it in water, keep it dry till it heals. To mend a broken bone, too, we must follow sequential steps. Imagine you have an ankle fracture. Now you wouldn't wear a cast—which will repair your bone in the correct alignment—and go for a walk when you are still healing, right?

Without following the sequential steps, the healing will be compromised. In the same manner, the sequential steps and tasks mentioned throughout this book are important for healing. Doing them in an unstructured manner will not produce the desired effect.

The key is to be sequential.

When I healed myself of rheumatoid arthritis, my body's ability to do extreme exercise was limited. But when I went back to learn yoga professionally, this ability had increased because my body had continuously been nourished so it could repair. Along with the process of sequentially nourishing myself, I also had some other positive effects. My ageing was slower, leading to reduced disease activity and no lifestyle diseases even though I have a family history of heart disease. I beat my genetics with my positive lifestyle.

My mind was in a state of conflict because I was carrying the baggage of memories of pain without those hurdles existing. The conflict was further compounded because of inputs from those around me. But the moment I made up my mind, my body listened to me. And that is what we must remember—making up your mind is the most powerful blessing nature has given us.

THE BODY IS A SLAVE OF THE MIND

Psychological stress is associated with greater risk for depression, heart disease and infectious diseases. Chronic psychological stress is associated with the body losing its ability to regulate the inflammatory response[46].

What is inflammation?

Inflammation is the immune system's response to injury, danger, and infection. It is the body's way of signalling the immune system to heal and repair damaged tissue, as well as defend itself against foreign invaders such as viruses and bacteria. When we are in a state of continuous stress and eat an inflammatory diet, inflammation levels in the form of blood markers become raised and can trigger lifestyle and inflammatory diseases, autoimmune diseases, and cancer. Inflammation is partly regulated by the hormone cortisol and when cortisol is not allowed to serve this function, inflammation can get out of control[47].

The bodily manifestations of stress are in the form of raised inflammation levels in the blood reports. Patients at risk for heart disease have an elevated C-reactive protein (CRP). Overweight people or those with bad lipids have a high level of Interleukin-6 (IL-6). This inflammation marker is also high in those diagnosed with cancer metastasis. Those with a high inflammation will have unexplained chronically high ESR and CRP. These are physical manifestations of what will ultimately trigger disease.

While we have five vital organs that are essential for survival—brain, heart, kidneys, liver, and lungs—it is the brain that controls the body, receiving and sending signals to organs through the nervous system and via secreted hormones. Fear is controlled here, and the body is directed to do what the brain wants it to do within its reasonable capabilities of wear and tear. So often we read about cases of people who have been 'medical marvels', extremely severe cases where the spine has been crushed and doctors have stated that the person will never be able to walk. And because of the strength of the mind, that patient has defied doctors and walked.

The most revolutionary case is of *New York Times* bestselling author Dr Joe Dispenza who said that he employed meditation techniques and visualization to heal his broken spine. From a prognosis of never walking physically, he healed his body and is now living pain-free and teaching others his methods. He was interviewed in the documentary *HEAL*, an inspirational film on people with autoimmune, cancer, and mysterious diseases. A must-watch.

Understanding the human body is not just about anatomy. Only understanding at the level of anatomy means that we do not consider ourselves more than a machine or car. Without the backdrop of the brain controlling the body and the mind controlling the brain, our body can either succumb to disease, rust away, or defy all odds and emerge stronger, more energetic, and more capable.

And when the mind starts getting rusty, distracted, dispersed and uncaring of the body, it manifests on the body as well. Anything that is not in use does get creaky and stiff. In the absence of not using the body, disease can set in.

What's speeding up your body's ageing process?

Not using your body can accelerate the ageing process, making you vulnerable to lifestyle diseases and cancer. How? It's because of the following connections which seemingly most people are unable to make:

1. You are immersed in work and have no gratitude for the fact that you have a physically able body. You're so distracted that you stop using your body.

2. If you do not use your body regularly with movement, circulation is impacted.

3. If there is poor circulation, oxygen and nutrients are not efficiently distributed throughout the body and organs, including the heart.

4. Due to lack of circulation, the metabolic rate dips, leading to a sluggish thyroid, compromised calorie-burning capabilities, and fat storage.

5. When the thyroid is impacted, the endocrine system gets impacted, leading to hormonal fluctuations which can be accompanied by weight gain, hypothyroidism, risk of hormonal diseases, and raised cortisol levels, leading to inflammation.

6. Low oxygen levels and lesser nutrients compromise the digestive system's ability to digest food, functioning of the heart, and functioning of the liver in releasing toxins. All these can compromise your ability to expel toxins and reduce lung capacity. The lungs need a certain amount of oxygen and carbon dioxide exchange on a regular basis to function well. Low movement will mean low oxygen.

7. The heart is impacted due to lower oxygen and nutrients; the lungs are impacted due to poor exchange of gases; and the liver is impacted due to slow release of toxins, making it sluggish.

8. The digestive system is impacted, leading to low absorption of nutrients, compromising the immune system further. There was already lesser circulation of nutrients due to inactivity, over and above that, absorption also reduces. Hence the immune system weakens.

The amount of time a person sits during the day is associated with a higher risk of heart disease, diabetes, cancer, and death, regardless of regular exercise, according to a review study published in January 2015 in the *Annals of Internal Medicine*.

This weakens the immune system and increases inflammation, leading to the above listed risks. All you did was sit in one place and focus on your work, your laptop. This work, ironically, will be taken away from you if your health is compromised. Organizations do not have time or patience for employees who have compromised outputs for work. So, the very work for which you compromised your health will no longer be there unless you focus on your health along with your work. Too much of work, sitting or too much of physical activity and over-exercising, both will negatively impact you.

The body needs balance.

And this is where our body is like the Earth we live on. As humans ravage the Earth, misuse, and abuse its resources, nature lashes back with earthquakes, pandemics, floods, and other natural disasters. Whether it is nature or our body, upsetting the balance will cause a backlash. Sustainable living is balanced living and has benefits not just for the Earth but also us. Growing or eating organic means lesser load of toxins for us and the earth; using frugality in consumption reduces the burden of production on farmers, and when the supply is in sync with the demand there's no need for adulteration of any kind. It also teaches us, as human beings, to balance the mind and body when we consume less, eat less, spend less, and appreciate more.

2

The Healing Benefits of Grounding

I remember when we were children, during heavy exam pressure, we were told to go walk on the grass to freshen up our brains so that we could absorb more. That is earthing or grounding.

Today, science has found data around why it is good for us even though we have known for centuries that it is beneficial. We all know that the Earth has a conductive surface, proven by electrical earthing used for plugs and switches to make an appliance safer. The earth is a conductor for protecting us from electrical shocks. For us human beings, who are made up of millions of cells, earthing (also known as grounding) refers to our contact with the Earth's surface electrons by walking barefoot outside or sitting, working or sleeping indoors, which transfers the energy from the ground into the body.

If antioxidants from a plant can seep into the human body, so can antioxidants and minerals from the earth. Our skin is our largest organ and the surface of the skin absorbs both positivity and negativity. We have heard of people getting poisoned through gas exposure; they inhaled it as much as their skin absorbed it. Similarly, we also absorb the minerals in the fresh air, ground, and from the grass we walk on. Earthing benefits include better sleep, reduced pain, and inflammation and this can be achieved by walking barefoot outside or sitting, working, or sleeping indoors connected to conductive systems that transfer the Earth's electrons from the ground into the body.

Integrative research has revealed that electrically conductive contact of our body with the surface of the Earth (grounding or earthing) produces anti-inflammatory effects on healing us[48]. In fact, photographic images documented the accelerated improvement in reduction of inflammation, healing of an eight-month-old, non-healing open wound suffered by an 84-year-old diabetic woman.

But Narender Sharma hasn't heard of earthing or grounding. And yet, she is reaping the benefits of it. Every morning, at 7 a.m., you will catch her singing one of her favourite songs, barefoot in her garden, watering her plants. At 72, she can stand for an hour, she walks her dog and is a working woman. This fiercely independent and vivacious young woman has a full day ahead of her as the principal of a school in New Delhi. Even her daughter says that she is still the same firebrand and age has not dulled her shine. She exercises five days a week, consumes vegetables every day and has not repeated a single sari in her entire life! Her verve for life is high. The only health issue she has ever had, which she takes medications for, is her thyroid which was a postmenopausal development. Unlike other (even younger) thyroid patients who experience brain fog, Narender ensures that her brain stays active by learning different courses, even today. She did a course with NIIT recently on computer science basics and MS office and took a course to improve her spoken English. Her continuous energy drives her to volunteer at old-age homes, a blind school for girls, Adarshila Cancer Hospital, and Hobbit camp to help orphaned girls and widows and essential service workers in her colony. She has also undertaken tree plantation drives around her school and home spaces.

In her spare time, you will find her in her little garden, humming an old romantic Hindi movie song. Born and brought up in Kuala Lumpur, she came to India at the age of 17. Her father was in the Indian National Army (INA) and her outgoing and strong nature made her a wonderful NCC cadet who took part in the Republic Day parade when she was 19. She became the hockey captain of her college team and president of the literacy group, and she won the popular Ms Fresher title. Even today, she epitomizes freshness. Her quality of life is enviable. Interestingly, she takes a reasonable amount of supplementation as well. Between the antioxidants from her food, her supplements, and the earthing in her garden, this 72-year-old vibrant woman has kept her youthful sprightliness intact.

So, what makes her tick and stay youthful? I would say it is a combination of the antioxidants that seep into her feet combined with the antioxidants in her vegetables, supplements, and neuroplasticity. Let us understand antioxidants from the earth and neuroplasticity in detail.

EARTHING AND NEUROPLASTICITY

Neuroplasticity is the brain's ability to modify its connections and function in response to environmental demands. It is an important input for the learning process. As we age, this ability declines, and like every other part of the body, our brain also starts getting slower. Unless, of course, we keep the brain agile just like our body. Regular brain exercises have been shown to maintain or increase neuroplasticity in older people as well.

In people with accelerated ageing—and I know a lot of middle-aged people who are going through this—slowing down of the brain happens much earlier, either due to mental lethargy or disease-driven brain fog. We start forgetting things, experience an inability to do normal tasks and so many of us shrug it off saying that we are growing older. But it is not true. The brain can be kept young and active as long as we are alive and breathing. In fact, people who have sharper memories and higher alertness levels are healthier, survive deadly diseases, and demonstrate a much better quality of everyday living. The more we keep our brain alive and intact, the higher our quality of life will be. The brain will remain resourceful in making sure that we have our optimum energy, we work till the end and have deeper social bonds. And the simple act of learning new tasks sequentially can keep this neuroplasticity alive.

Narender keeps her mind curious for knowledge. This curiosity has driven her to keep the brain neurons active and sharp by relearning—like she did the computer science and language courses at this age—and that increases neuroplasticity. She did a computer science course at the age of 72.

A person facing low brain energy at the age of 45 or 50, due to accelerated ageing or disease, can keep it alive by something as simple as doing crossword puzzles, learning a new language or doing a course on something which is totally different from what their profession, education or career has been about till now. People on heavy medications, those who have been through chemotherapy treatments and autoimmune patients experience brain ageing much more and can overcome this by learning new tasks.

So how do these tasks impact our brain?

Neuroplasticity is very strong as we learn to map our surroundings using the senses. As we grow older, plasticity decreases to stabilize what we have already learnt. This stabilization is partly controlled by a neurotransmitter called gamma-Aminobutyric acid (GABA), which inhibits neuronal activity[49]. Of course, this discovery has given rise to companies selling GABA supplements touting it as brain food.

But the best benefits of neuroplasticity being intact will always be the long road—you must train your brain to make new neural pathways by ditching old memory. So, if you are an electronics engineer, do a course in painting. It is completely different from what you have ever done, and you do not have any stored memory of it. The new memories that are formed in the process of learning how to paint will be making new neural pathways which, in turn, make your brain agile. It's very simple if you equate it to your body. People who do not exercise have sore joints, slower movement, and low balance. Using your body makes your body strong, more balanced, and younger. Using your brain has the same effect on your brain.

And the brain controls your ageing so if your brain is young, it will push your body to remain young.

A simpler way to keep your brain young is to walk on the grass, on the beach, in the garden, barefoot. That not only refreshes the brain because of the absorption of antioxidants from the earth but also reduces inflammation levels in various parts of the body. And we have already learnt that inflammation is the root cause that triggers all lifestyle diseases.

Now who would have imagined that science would back this simple habit followed by people for centuries.

3

Understanding Accelerated Physical Ageing

Very simply put, if you are ageing faster than your chronological age, you have accelerated ageing. Why does this happen?

Our chronological age is irreversible but our biological age, which is dependent on how we live, can easily be lower. Consider this—the damage to your cells and tissues caused by daily activities, stress, and wear and tear can be repaired by a healthy lifestyle and eight hours of sleep. However, if you don't repair daily, this damage accumulates, causing accelerated ageing. All because you did not give your body the time and space to repair via proper nourishment and sleep. Hence, your biological age will increase and that is what causes premature ageing.

It is like your financial status.

You can spend and overspend and live on credit till you reach the stage of debt. Accelerated ageing is debt. The human body and mind need a certain time and input to repair any damage at a physical, emotional, and neurological level on a *daily* basis. There will be damage because the physical body is being used, the brain and mind are labouring and they need to be rested, cleansed, and rejuvenated every day. When this repair work doesn't occur daily, there is a deficit that builds up; it can happen over a few years. And that is when diseases we were meant to have as part of the natural degeneration process of ageing start to happen at a young age.

Simply put, if you buy a new car and don't look after it, in four years, you will have to junk the car. However, the human mind and body are much more complex than a car, any machine, or a broken financial state.

Nurturing via holistic nutrition must be daily because the damage is happening daily.

The normal ageing process also makes energy deficit, triggering diseases. Our cells extract energy from nutrients. Every time we inhale, the blood transports oxygen from our lungs to our cells' mitochondria, where it is used to convert the nutrients in our food into a form of energy that the body can use. Problems with this process, called cell respiration, have been linked to numerous conditions, from rare genetic diseases to diabetes, cancer, Parkinson's disease, and the normal ageing process. For cell respiration to function properly, it needs proteins synthesized outside and then imported into the mitochondria, and proteins synthesized within the mitochondria themselves from their own DNA (mtDNA). It has long been known that an accumulation of harmful mutations of mtDNA can cause premature ageing. This premature ageing can stop when positive epigenetic changes (read lifestyle changes) repair response of our DNA.

Activating our anti-ageing gene

We all have an anti-ageing protein or gene in our body called SIRT1 which controls ageing. And if we can activate this gene via the specific healthy lifestyle given, we are changing our response to the speed of ageing.

This repair work daily is not very difficult. It can be fulfilled with holistic nutrition, and it becomes a powerful preventive tool to give a quality of life that slows down ageing and risk of diseases. And reducing your risk to get diseases means lower costs, higher agility, and higher energy levels to be able to do everyday tasks more efficiently and live a life that is enviable.

What is the impact of accelerated ageing on the human body? Let's look at it in detail below.

Your mood is off. Mostly Try and remember the last time you had a stomach upset or a viral fever. You were not feeling good, your energy levels were low and if somebody tried to push you into doing something you didn't want to, you snapped. Now, if you don't have an illness or disease and you are still in that state, it is indicative of something going wrong inside which is yet undiagnosed. When you're not well, and you don't know about it because it has not yet manifested into a physical symptom like a heart attack, hypertension or type 2 diabetes, the best way is to analyse your moods. A person who is in balance physically and mentally, is often going to have mature and even moods. Here, we are not talking about a one-off response like a burst of anger. We are talking about people who *used to be fine*, but now are consistently in a poor mood, don't see the positive side in most situations or spread the sarcasm more than the sunshine. If that behaviour is continued and consistent, it is the most prominent sign of disease and accelerated ageing.

Your inflammation levels rise As explained earlier, inflammation levels are measured by markers in our blood and they predict the rate of disease activity. Even when you feel absolutely healthy but have had some kind of physical or emotional deficit in the repair work, your inflammation markers like CRP and ESR will be high. If there is a logical rise in ESR levels, it is usually due to an infection or allergy. However, if you have not experienced any infection or allergy and are feeling healthy and have been feeling 'fine', defined as 'absence of disease', then you get into a state of chronic inflammation. You may have symptoms that you are not acknowledging, like low moods, poor energy or not waking up fresh.

Chronic inflammation means that your ESR and CRP are consistently high and remain so for long periods of time in the absence of any infection, allergy, or disease diagnosis. They are the best predictors of inflammatory diseases including cancer. Get them checked.

Your risk of getting lifestyle diseases is extremely high Naturally, if you have chronic inflammation you may be sitting on disease activity inside. You may not be aware of it because you did not get any blood tests done. There was nothing 'wrong' with you except a bit of stress here or there. So, you don't know how to get into a preventive situation, and it is not till you physically have symptoms that you will go to a doctor for a diagnosis. By this time, you have already reached a reactive mode to your gross body's symptoms rather than listening to the symptoms presented by your subtle body.

What are the gross and subtle bodies? They both reside inside you. In yogic teachings, the subtle body is one of the three bodies that together constitute a human existence. It is also known as sukshma sharira or astral body. The other two bodies are the physical body (gross body) and the causal body (the most complex—the seed which connects the other two bodies). In the Bhagavad Gita, the subtle body is described as a confluence of mind, intellect, and ego, and it controls the physical.

As a holistic human being, if you are in touch with yourself and aware of your body even in two of its forms—gross and subtle—you are able to identify the symptoms of wear and tear before a health crisis occurs. Subtle body always gives signs for inflammation but if the subtle energy is not activated in a lot of us, these symptoms are not acknowledged. People aware of the subtle body are more in touch with their here and now. Being overwhelmed, stressed, tired, overeating, eating too many carbohydrates, and a sedentary lifestyle suppresses the symptoms the subtle body is trying to give us. It is like living in a stupor; we are a complete physical and emotional being, but we are not aware of our self. Mindful living can easily break this stupor.

I have known people at the age of 30 with type 2 diabetes, high cholesterol, and fatty liver who refused to acknowledge that they could get these conditions. It was only through extensive questioning that I saw the symptoms and pushed them for blood test reports because I suspected the disease. And that is how the diagnosis happened. If they had continued to live like this, early diagnosis would not have been possible to contain the damage.

Your day-to-day life gets impacted An inflammatory environment inside the body means your energy levels are low, your brain is functioning at a slower pace and even after eight hours of sleep you are not fresh. At a physical level, this is going to impact your work (because your output is going to be compromised), your relationships (because you're not going to have the energy to enjoy simple and loving tasks with loved ones), and, finally, make you feel pessimistic about your present and future. This pessimism can very quickly turn into chronic anxiety, depression and manifest in unexplained tremors, sudden weight gain or weight loss, substance abuse (which includes junk food), etc. All of these will make you age even faster and increase risk of lifestyle diseases.

Your medical visits rise So many of us go from one symptom to the other and get treated for those symptoms. Acidity? Antacids. Palpitations? Anti-anxiety drugs. Insomnia? Sleeping pill. Instead of going to the root cause and eliminating the symptom, these ad hoc measures suppress the underlying inflammation and problems. This can lead to late diagnosis of the disease, causing more suffering.

Whether you are in a country like India, which is not completely covered by medical insurance, or in any developed part of the world where everyone is covered by insurance, it is extremely distressing and inconvenient to keep visiting the doctor or hospital. Even if you are covered by medical insurance, sometimes you wait months to get an appointment or treatment because the medical system is so overburdened already. During this waiting time, the distress you cause to your body and the continuing spread of your disease is only driving you to a point of no return.

Ill-health increases the vicious cycle of fear and anxiety, and the joy of everyday living disappears. The only certainty in life is that we will age and die. But there is that period in between which is meant to be enjoyed.

It's called life.

4

Life Is Like a Road Trip

When we set out on a road trip, we pack picnic snacks, some water, maybe a flask of tea or coffee, a blanket for those sitting behind, especially kids. And a playlist of songs everybody can enjoy. Are we then getting into the vehicle thinking *only* about our destination? No. While we have the destination in mind, our immediate focus shifts to how to make the road journey enjoyable. There is the countryside, breathtaking views, a few rocky paths, a traffic jam, animals crossing the road, stops at dhabas to experience local food, visits to the washroom and so much more.

Just like a road trip, life is full of such breaks, traffic jams, urgent visits to the washroom, but it is also full of enjoying the picnic in the car, soaking in nature while driving, listening to your favourite song and snuggling into a blanket, biting into delicious food made by somebody else, stretching your legs … All these joys make the journey special.

This experience can be enhanced so much more if we are in balance and give the right inputs to nourish ourselves because that heightens our sense of everyday joy.

Balancing your body and mind ensures that you prevent, manage or even reverse diseases. A lifestyle promoting anti-inflammatory inputs reduces inflammation, lowering disease activity and making disease parameters and symptoms disappear.

Take the case of Sameer Anjaria. As a senior telecom leader who travelled for work twenty days a month, Sameer lived out of guesthouses, had high cholesterol and type 2 diabetes. At the age of 45, he decided that he wanted to change his quality of life and got in touch with me. Within three months, not only did his cholesterol levels and HbA1c come back to normal range but his energy levels were extremely high, he lost weight, and overall, was experiencing a better quality of life.

Instead of suppressing his symptoms with medications, he made his mind *speak* to his body to repair it. And his body listened to his mind.

This miracle of repair does many things—it increases our energy, makes us mentally sharp and physically agile and gives us the ability to enjoy every day without waking up tired or with pains. And the road trip of life can only be appreciated when the state of body and mind are fresh and energetic.

5

The Right Physical Balance

In tangible terms, if you nurture and nourish yourself, your immediate life also improves. So, what can you expect? Let's examine some physical outcomes. Everybody around you is telling you that you need to exercise and eat right to have the following goals:

1. **Be lean** This is the biggest burden we carry because of the public perception of a body image as well as the foundation of good health being driven by being in weight-range. The latter is true.

2. **Prevent diseases** Including cancer, that word which causes fear in our minds.

3. **Manage existing diseases better** Even if you are on the most toxic drugs, side effects of these medications can be drastically reduced, strengthening your gut and immune system so that your dependency on medications disappears over a period of time. All factors influence our health, wellness, and disease, including mind, spirit, and community, as well as the body. The correct use of conventional and alternative methods

facilitates the body's instinctive healing response. Understanding which one to use when becomes the key. Western medicine is emergency medicine—in ninety per cent of the cases it needs to be used when the body has reached a distressful situation. But for lifestyle diseases, this can be prevented or managed better by integrating holistic nutrition to balance physical and emotional inputs on a consistent basis.

4. **Reverse diseases** This is what I specialize in. When I take on a patient, I don't take them on to help them manage their condition; my focus and aim is to help them reduce disease activity and inflammation levels to such an extent that the causes of the disease start disappearing[50]. I have achieved this consistently over time with my patients since 2008 and before that with myself.

5. **Experience positivity** This is the highest impact of being in a good state of physical and emotional health. When you are unwell, you're irritable, crabby, low on patience, forgetful or have a gloomier outlook towards your life and future. Decision-making is poor and compromised. But with good health comes positivity and balanced moods. You may blame your impatience on too much work and worry, but when there is harmony and balance between mind and body, the same work can be streamlined and completed in a more efficient manner (and faster!) because your brain is functioning at a faster capacity. This leaves you with more time for yourself and loved ones as well as to pursue your interests.

Achieving this balance is a form of self-respect.

At the age of 22, Saharanpur-based Gulshan Phutela was already a business partner. He was the youngest of four partners who ran a shop. Around this time, he also met a sadhu whom he spent a full month with. He lived with the sadhu, did yoga, ate with him, and learnt the meaning of life from this wise man. And the one thing that stuck with him was what this sadhu repeatedly told him:

'Your body is a gift from God. Treat it like a gift, nurture it and look after it.'

Under his tutelage, Gulshan learnt yoga and has been practising it every day. At 79, he doesn't have any lifestyle or degenerative diseases, is not on any medication, and lives a full life. 'My body is God's kripa,' he says.

There were other ways that he was wise beyond his years as a young man, maybe due to the physical and emotional balance inculcated by the sadhu. Just when he got married, he was thrilled that he had a very beautiful wife. 'Everybody loves beauty, don't they?' he asked me with a mischievous glint in his eyes.

He would leave the house at 7 a.m. and return by 8 p.m. One day, before they had children, his wife asked him, 'Why did you marry me if you don't even have time to spend with me?'

This question hit Gulshan hard. He went back to his business partners and negotiated a deal for working from 11 a.m. to 6 p.m. Since he was hard-working and efficient, his partners relented. This extra time was spent in romance, bonding and building a strong relationship with his wife. Then they had children. Now, he wanted to spend time with his children and holiday with them. So, he went back to his partners and told them that he wanted to take thirty days off every year. This could be thirty days at a stretch or ten days every quarter.

'My partners were in their mid 50s while I was still in my 20s. I wanted to travel, spend time with my family, watch my children grow up, whereas they had already done all this.' His partners discussed amongst themselves and came back and gave him an offer—they asked him to reduce his partnership stake by two per cent. Each one of the four partners had a twenty-five per cent stake in the business, and this would mean reducing his stake to twenty-three per cent, and they would divide the two per cent amongst the three of them.

Gulshan knew a good chartered accountant, and he sought his advice. The chartered accountant asked him to jump at the opportunity; this was an extremely fair deal.

And that was how Gulshan's quality of life was sealed. 'I was never driven by money,' he told me. Having said that, he was prudent enough to not only earn well but also save up to have a wonderful old age. The family began to travel frequently and finally decided that they wanted to have a summer home in Mussoorie. Now, in their sunset years, Gulshan and his wife spend the summers in Mussoorie where the weather is cool and pleasant with less pollution. 'I don't like being in the air conditioner, and I also save money,' he admits. 'Extreme summers spent in Mussoorie mean less electricity bills and more enjoyment.'

All through the Zoom interview, I was marvelling at this man. His daily schedule is reflective of what the sadhu taught

him, and his focus is in keeping his health and balance intact.
His daily schedule is as below:

- *He wakes up at 6 a.m.* 'I need to rev up my circulation as soon as I wake up, so on the bed itself I do twenty exercises of one minute each.' After that, he prays for twenty minutes. Post the prayer, he walks barefoot on his beautiful lawn, drinks lots of water. And then he goes to the bathroom to clear his bowels. 'I always take a minute for bowel movements, no more,' he admits, dismissing the need to take reading material. If digestion is strong, the job is done immediately, he says. I like him so much!
- *8 a.m.* He and his wife both have white pumpkin juice, again to clear the stomach. After that, it's time for yoga followed by 'sunlight bath' and one hour of body massage.
- *9.30 a.m.* He has his bath.
- *10 a.m.* A very light breakfast.
- *11 a.m.* Salad, which consists of one full plate seasonal veggies.
- *12 noon* A bowl of seasonal fruits.
- *2 p.m.* Lunch is two rotis made from atta (flour) with chopped green leaves for easy digestion. A portion of vegetables with less spice is his accompaniment.
- *4 p.m.* Salted limewater.
- *5–7 p.m.* This is his recreational time at the local club. 'We have games, table tennis, cards, swimming; I walk around and catch up with friends every day,' he says.

- *7.30 p.m.* He reaches home and dinner is primarily fruit and sprouts. Even though he goes to the club every day, he doesn't eat out much. 'I don't take white flour. As we age, we must change our diet because at a young age you can digest anything, but with age digestion weakens,' he says. And then his enjoyment: whenever he does go out with friends, is two small 30 ml drinks of vodka.

'Anything in limit is fine. Ghee will be unhealthy if you exceed limits. Six months ago, I stopped milk products. I saw this video where it was explained that milk is for the calf. It is not made for humans by God. Chemicals, hormones, impurities are put into it. So, if you understand it, you won't consume it. My body is God's kripa, why should I make it impure?' he says.

Gulshan and I get into a discussion around milk and milk products and he asks me if I agree with what he just said. Definitely, I share with him that this is exactly my philosophy as well and even if we are consuming out of a personal choice, milk and milk products like any other animal protein should not be more than five per cent of our daily lives and it should be from a pure and organic source.

I ask him for his words of wisdom for all of us and he says, 'Too much greed; money is driving us. Without health, money is of no use. Look after your health, your body, as that is the vehicle you have and don't dismiss the importance of sleep because that is what is going to repair your body.'

The biggest impact of his lifestyle is that he has influenced his family towards the path of good health. His two daughters were gushing all over him just before I began the interview and had admiration in their eyes. Both have chosen the path of becoming healers because their father's lifestyle inspired them to stay healthy and help others be healthy. Their father's jovial mood creates a harmonious environment at home, leading those around him to push for the happiness quotient much more.

The balance that Gulshan demonstrates in everything helped him achieve a state of no disease even at the age of 79. It is easy for all of us to dismiss his lifestyle and say that we don't have this kind of time and it is not practical. But we must remember that Gulshan has been following this lifestyle of moderation and balance since the age of 22 and that is the reason that he has enjoyed the journey of life. At a young age, he balanced out his work hours so that he could spend time with loved ones. He saved prudently and spent less. This helped him stay conscious of frugality and kept his mind and body nimble.

His wisdom beyond his years came because of the early days of exposure to the sadhu and his learnings. And so, physical and emotional balance lead to wise decision-making, stable moods, and a life which had the balance of work, family time, and me time.

As a businessman, Gulshan could achieve this balance because he did not fear asking his partners for what he desired. Whether you are a businessperson or a salaried person, asking never hurts. And when you verbalize what you want, very often the universe conspires to give it to you. Even when you are praying to God, you need to ask the higher power what you want. Hence, fulfilment of all desires starts by asking, manifesting what you want. Go on, ask your boss for just a little bit of free time or coming in one hour late every day to work. That one hour can be utilized in sleeping late and exercising on alternate days.

Just one hour and you would have achieved the beautiful balance your body needs. Ask, manifest.

6

Gentle Yoga Schedule

Yoga is one of the four pillars of holistic nutrition. The four pillars are:

1. Vegetables and fruits in every meal for those anti-inflammatory cancer-fighting nutrients.
2. Breath work every day. To calm the fluctuations of an agitated brain.
3. Gentle yoga thrice a week. To bring peace and agility to every joint and increase circulation so that the nutrients can be absorbed by every part of us.
4. Sleep. To repair and rejuvenate the damage of everyday living and release latent stress and inflammation.

I call this my VBYS. It is my new acronym of the rainbow to achieve good health.

It isn't for no reason that there's been a global movement around the benefits of yoga as a mind–body exercise. Even though the mass acceptability of yoga in India came after people in the West started following it, the benefits of yoga and the improvements it can demonstrate when combined with nutrition are timeless. I have already shared with you the kind of foods that help the mind stay calm; when you combine that kind of holistic nutrition with gentle yoga, the miracle of healing begins. And that is why yoga forms one of the four pillars of holistic nutrition.

Yoga is adaptive to our health issues and limitations. Let us go far back—the yoga guru BKS Iyengar was stricken by the influenza pandemic in his village and even though he survived, as a child, he suffered from malnutrition, tuberculosis, malaria, and many other illnesses. At the age of fifteen, he was sent to learn yoga to gain some strength. And like all of us learning yoga, he too had a rocky start with his teacher because the latter did not believe that the tough practices of Hatha Yoga, which focuses on the physical body becoming stronger, could be done by this thin spindly boy.

But of course, the power of the mind is stronger than the weak body. Iyengar's teacher, Tirumalai Krishnamacharya, was a strict Hatha Yoga teacher and would punish the little boy by starving him if the asanas were not perfected. Iyengar not only endured this but grew up to revive modern Hatha Yoga across India and the world.

But something more happened.

Driven by the memory of the pains of being malnourished and physically weak as a child, Iyengar developed a form of yoga people with pains could do. And so, Restorative Yoga was invented by Iyengar for people who could not do the traditional form of yoga due to physical limitations. This form of yoga uses props like belts, cushions, blankets, and blocks to aid people in restoring themselves from illnesses. The reason it is so successful today is because it was invented by someone who had been through this pain and understood the human body in relieving the pain.

Today, yoga is for everyone. Whether you have learnt via the principles of Maharishi Patanjali with Ashtanga Yoga or Swatmaramji's Hatha Yoga or any other school, the benefits of yoga translate to calming the fluctuations of the mind by conquering the body.

There are eight forms of yoga:

1. Ashtanga Yoga
2. Hatha Yoga
3. Mantra Yoga
4. Bhakti Yoga
5. Kundalini Yoga
6. Karma Yoga
7. Kriya Yoga
8. Swara Yoga

With increasing health issues, these traditional forms of yoga have been adapted to help people overcome health issues and increase quality of life. While Restorative Yoga is for those looking at reducing chronic pain, fatigue, and stress levels, especially people recovering from illnesses including cancer and autoimmune conditions, Yin Yoga is for girls and women suffering from hormonal issues.

Yin Yoga was invented in the early 1970s by Pauli Zinc. This is the slow-pace form combining traditional Indian and Chinese postures. The Chinese and Indian yoga philosophy is similar: meridians in the subtle body are the same as nadis in Hatha Yoga. In Yin Yoga, poses apply moderate stress to connective tissues and the approach is more meditative, helping ease hormonal distress in women. With the entire female human population sitting on a hormonal storm, Yin Yoga has shown clinical hormone-pacifying results and relief in symptoms.

Whichever form of yoga you start with, the key is to practise it daily and gently urge your mind and body to reach just a little higher every single day.

Yoga chittavriti nirodhah (Calm the fluctuations of the mind)

The purpose of yoga is to calm the fluctuations of the mind.

The next few pages are for those of you who have led a sedentary life, not been introduced to yoga, and even those who go to the gym or do strenuous exercise. The benefits of gentle yoga in reducing stress levels and increasing flexibility will be amazing.

Follow these poses to start training your body to get ready for the next level of healing: where it is strong, balanced, and disease-free.

Daily yoga schedule

Do remember, you don't have to be worried about bending yourself out of shape by copying extremely flexible people; do your own thing as per your own body's capability. But be unhurried in your practice.

Step 1: Rev up the circulation

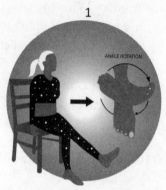

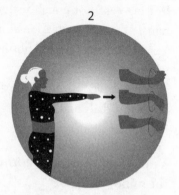

Sit straight in a chair, stretch your right leg in front, and rotate your right ankle clockwise, *slowly*, 10 times. Then repeat with your left ankle.

Stand up straight, with arms in front. Rotate right wrist clockwise 10 times, and then anti-clockwise, *slowly*. Do the same with left wrist.

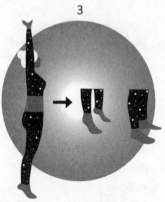

Tadasana: Stretch fully, raising your arms above your head, standing on your toes. Go up and down from toes to heels *slowly*, 10 times. Relax.

4

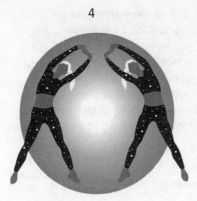

Stretch your waist by bending while standing straight. First the left side, hold for 10 seconds. Then the right side, hold for 10 seconds. Repeat 10 times for each side.

5

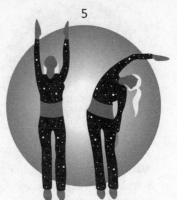

Stretch your waist by bending while standing straight. First the left side, hold for 10 seconds. Then the right side, one hand up, one down, hold for 10 seconds. Repeat 10 times for each side.

6

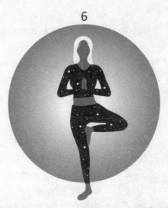

Modified Vrikshasana: Stand straight and balance your right leg with your left toe touching your knee. Hold for 10 seconds or as long as you can balance. Repeat with your left leg. Do thrice for each leg. Use a wall for support initially.

Step 2: Fill in some oxygen and gratitude

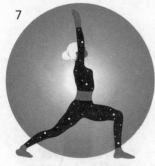

7

Warrior (Veerbhadrasana)
Warrior 1 is a natural pose that gives your back a nice stretch as it strengthens your core, thighs, and buttocks. It fills your chest with oxygen as you inhale. This is a calming position that promotes clarity in thinking and mental peace.

Warrior 1 (Veerbhadrasana 1)
Step 1: Begin in a standing position with your feet brought together and your hands by your side.
Step 2: Extend your right leg forward as you push your left leg backward, similar to a lunge movement.
Step 3: Slightly turn your midsection so that you are facing your bent right knee.
Step 4: Give your body added support by slightly turning your left leg.
Step 5: Inhale as you raise your body up from your knees.
Step 6: Slowly stretch your arms upwards as you bend your back to form a slight arch.
Step 7: Remain in this position for 15-30 seconds, breathe normally.
Step 8: Slowly break the pose by exhaling and straightening your right knee. Push off your right leg and allow yourself to come back gently into the original pose.
Step 9: Repeat with the opposite leg.

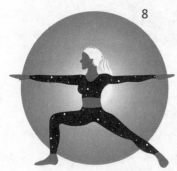

8

Warrior 2 (Veerbhadrasana 2)
Step 1: Follow the same steps as before, but instead of raising your hands above your head, extend them outwards from your torso, inhaling deeply.
Step 2: Turn your head so that you are facing your right leg. Hold for fifteen seconds.
Step 3: Repeat with your left leg.

9

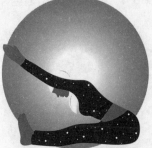

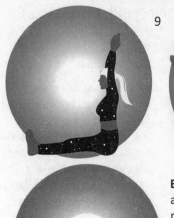

Back stretch: Slowly stretch your arms and lie down as much as possible on your knees as per the illustration *without overstretching*. Go with your body's capability, not the illustration. Breathe normally and hold for 20 seconds. Release. Repeat 3 times. This exercise is wonderful for female hormones, spine issues, and belly. Increase hold time to 1 minute in a few weeks.

10

Spine twist: Lie down on the floor, with hands below your head. Inhale deeply, rotate your spine from your waist for both legs to the right, hold for 10 seconds, then exhale while bringing your legs back to the centre. Inhale and rotate to the left and hold for 10 seconds. Repeat 3 times for each side. Increase hold time to 1 minute in a few weeks. This exercise stretches and strengthens the spine. It is a must-do, twice-a-day exercise for those who sit for long hours at a stretch.

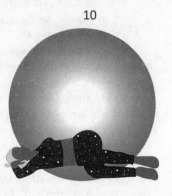

Step 4: Strengthen the spine and release stress

11

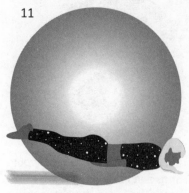

Modified Locust Pose (Salabhasana)

Lie down on your stomach, with your legs fully stretched. Stay in that position for 10 seconds. Release. Repeat 3 times. Increase hold time to 1 minute in a few weeks. This exercise relieves stress, fatigue, and strengthens the spine.

12

Bridge (Setu Bandha Sarvangasana)

Start by lying on your back. Slide your feet up so that your ankles are below your knees and your feet are flat on the floor. Squeeze your butt muscles as you raise your hips towards the ceiling. Your weight should be on your shoulders. Hold 10 seconds. Increase hold time to 1 minute in a few weeks. Repeat thrice. This exercise releases stress, balances hormones, stretches the spine, the legs, and improves digestion.

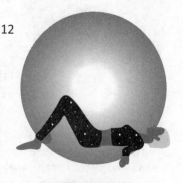

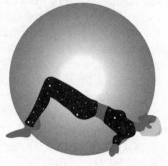

Continued ... Step 4: Strengthen the spine and release stress

13   14

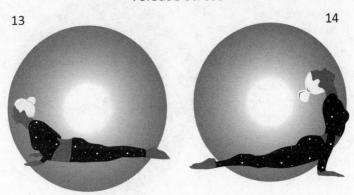

Cobra Pose (Bhujangasana)

The cobra pose is a multi-muscle workout. It is great for those with hypothyroidism. It strengthens both the spine and the upper body.

Step 1: Practise only with hand pressure (illustration on the left). Do not stretch more than you can or you may injure your back.
Step 2: Only increase pressure on hands and lift up after you gain strength. Otherwise, continue with step 1.

How to do it:
Step 1: Start by lying stomach down on the mat.
Step 2: Stretch your legs away from your body as you pull your arms in under your shoulders with your palms on the side as shown above.
Step 3: Allow your toes and chin to touch the floor.
Step 4: Inhale deep and slow as you thrust your upper body and chest upward.
Step 5: Hold the pose for 15–30 seconds and slowly exhale.
Step 6: Rest for 15 seconds.
Step 7: Repeat 5 times with a break in between each pose. Increase hold time to 1 minute in a few weeks.

Step 5: Improve digestion

Wind-easing Pose (Pavanamukthasan)

15

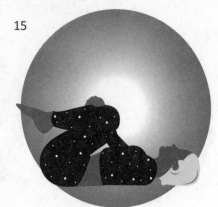

The wind-easing posture is a great pose for soothing lower back pain, strengthening your core, hips, and thighs. It has even been used to promote healthy pH levels and increase metabolism.

How to do it:

Step 1: Lie on your back with your legs stretched out, your heels touching each other, and your arms by your side.

Step 2: Exhale as you bend your knees and move them towards your chest.

Step 3: Hold your knees as you pull them closer into your body.

Step 4: Tighten your thighs and apply pressure to your abdominal muscles as you hold the position.

Step 5: Hold the position for 60–90 seconds as you breathe deliberately and deeply.

Step 6: Exhale and release your knees as you allow your arms to rest by your side.

Step 7: Repeat 5 times with a 15-second break between each pose.

You may pass wind, which is a good sign.

Step 6: Let go of anxiety

16

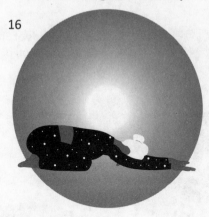

Child's Pose (Balasana)

1. Kneel on the floor with your toes together and your knees hip-width apart. Rest your palms on top of your thighs.
2. While exhaling, lower your torso between your knees. Extend your arms alongside your torso with your palms facing down. Relax your shoulders on the ground.
3. Rest in the pose for 30 seconds, build up to 5 minutes daily.

Child's Pose is relaxing because opening the hips and stretching the back relieves the tension caused by daily movements. By allowing you to breathe deeply, clean oxygen circulates in your body, restoring your energy. It also releases anxiety and helps you sleep better.

Step 7: Calm the mind with breath work

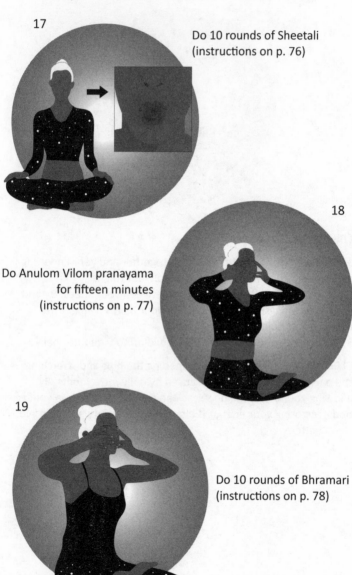

17

Do 10 rounds of Sheetali
(instructions on p. 76)

18

Do Anulom Vilom pranayama
for fifteen minutes
(instructions on p. 77)

19

Do 10 rounds of Bhramari
(instructions on p. 78)

Step 8: Open your heart with meditation

20

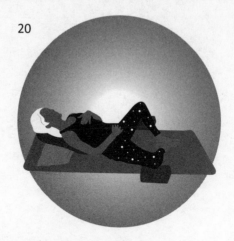

Supported Reclining Bound Angle Pose

Lie down in the position as shown in the above illustration with music on. Remain like this for 10 minutes.
This exercise has several benefits:

Stimulates abdominal organs like the ovaries and prostate gland, bladder, and kidneys.
Stimulates the heart and improves general circulation.
Stretches the inner thighs, groin, and knees.
Helps relieve the symptoms of stress, mild depression, menstruation, and menopause.
Aids sound sleep.

Part 4

The Learnings

They are alive. But the health gurus don't agree.

1

What the Ageless Have in Common

In total, I interviewed fifty-plus people for this book. What emerged wasn't what you have read in books, blogs, medical journals, and discourses from wellness gurus as the elixir for good health. They all talk about a unidimensional view for health, disease, quality of life, and longevity.

So, what are these elusive multidimensional parameters which we can learn from? And how do they match up to what science tells us?

I shared just a few of the journeys of these beautifully healthy people with you but each one has the following in common:

1. Eating a little, not too much.
2. Moderate exercise, not too much.
3. A dash of forbidden foods, not too much.
4. Spending time with nature.
5. Staying in touch.
6. Me time.
7. Being mentally active.
8. Positivity (which is a result of the above seven habits).

Now let's elaborate on all these, based on science.

EATING A LITTLE, NOT TOO MUCH

The benefits of satisfying eighty per cent of your hunger have been proven equally by almost every scientific experiment, clinical study, diet fads that work, and ancient texts of Ayurveda. Whether you look at intermittent fasting, which is becoming very popular because of its benefits, or the concept of 'akash' in Ayurveda, one of the interpretations of which is to leave your stomach just a little empty, eating less than your appetite leaves space in your stomach for the digestive juices to work more effectively. This increases absorption of nutrients and reduces the load on digestion. Continuously practising twenty per cent less food ensures digestive system repair. Once the gut starts healing, ninety per cent of diseases can be prevented or overcome quickly because, as we have seen, the gut and immune system are connected.

Reduced calorie intake of just twenty per cent less (not to be confused with starvation) has also been linked to activation of SIRT1, our anti-ageing gene, and has shown drastic reduction in ageing as well as onset of lifestyle and degenerative diseases. Lastly, benefits are a lessened risk of lifestyle diseases and cancer. Since obesity increases inflammation levels and risk of lifestyle diseases, just staying in your weight range, along with a moderate consumption of food, has been shown to reverse type 2 diabetes, accelerate weight loss, reduce risk of cancer, and keep joints agile.

Most of the people I interviewed ate either vegetables or fruits in every meal. The most potent anti-inflammatory and anti-cancer nutrients are found in these two and if you consistently consume them at every meal, they reduce side effects of anything else you are eating on your plate which could be potentially inflammatory. For example, Laurence eats a small dessert immediately after her dinner which is not recommended as a 'healthy' practice. However, she eats her vegetables and fruits across all meals. Her only indulgence is that small quantity of dessert (French women are known for small portion sizes) and often, that dessert ends up being dark chocolate which has antioxidants packed in it.

MODERATE EXERCISE, NOT TOO MUCH

Is somebody who goes to the gym healthy? What about someone who runs marathons? No, not necessarily. Excessive exercise causes oxidative stress and this stress is evident in the form of exercise-related injuries and suppressed immunity. Many marathon runners face rhinitis and frequent colds— when we put the body under extreme circumstances, the oxidative stress causes accelerated ageing. Many would argue with me about this, citing examples of healthy people running marathons. However, I have had many marathon runners coming to me with severe ankle issues, hardening of arteries, and chronic fatigue.

Doctors at the University of Maryland Medical Center found their 51-year-old doctor colleague who was the picture of good health—no cardiovascular risks, a marathon runner who had exercised vigorously each day for as many as thirty years—had just flunked a calcium screening scan of his heart. The researchers concluded that the physician's intense, long-term exercise regimen, coupled with a predisposition towards a type of hypertension, contributed to his cardiovascular disease. 'In this particular individual, we think that oxidative stress was an important contributor,' says the study's senior author, Michael Miller, MD, director of preventive cardiology at the University of Maryland Medical Center and associate professor of medicine at the University of Maryland School of Medicine. 'But we also found that this individual has exercise-induced hypertension, which is vastly underdiagnosed[51].

Exercise-induced hypertension is real.

On the other hand, a sedentary lifestyle can lead to accelerated stiffening of the muscle in the heart's left ventricle, the chamber that pumps oxygen-rich blood back out to the body. Sitting for too long causes as much oxidative stress as over-exercise.

Whether it is Gulshan, Steven, Ronnie or Laurence, everyone has had moderate exercise in the form of walks or yoga. Many of them do both with amazing results in the form of low disease activity and a healthy heart. Among most of the people I interviewed and the people that I treat, moderate, consistent, and balanced exercise does not cause oxidative stress. Rather, it reduces inflammation levels, anxiety, and regenerates neurons.

As we age, we begin to experience memory loss, brain fog, and balance issues. All these are addressed with consistent moderate exercise, which consists of moderate paced walks and gentle yoga. Exercise can reverse damage to sedentary, ageing hearts and help prevent risk of heart failure[52]. And heart disease patients who practise yoga in addition to aerobic exercise saw twice the reduction in blood pressure, body mass index (BMI), and cholesterol levels when compared to patients who practised either only yoga or only aerobic exercise[53].

So, what is moderate activity and how does it impact our DNA? Moderate activity would be forty-five minutes of brisk walking or thirty minutes of slow jogging, five days a week, along with minimum of two days of yoga (though my personal recommendation would be five!). This is the combination that increases telomere length, which demonstrates that it reduces the ageing process. According to a Brigham Young University study[54], the shortest telomeres came from sedentary people; those who had consistently high levels of physical activity had significantly longer telomeres.

With science backing regular moderate exercise, the key word is consistency, and it is possible to reduce ageing, mortality, and prolong life. This is because the heart and other organs will automatically reduce ageing activity if our telomeres are long[55].

Hence, exercise moderately, not too little, not too much.

SPENDING TIME WITH NATURE

After Ronnie recovered from the year-long lung oedema, his go-to place is that little garden with the peace lilies. For Steve, it is nature walks with his wife Andréa. For Laurence, it is the trees. For Narender, it's earthing.

For each one of them, there is an aspect of being closer to nature that calls out to them and makes them do just a little bit of gardening in their homes. In fact, gardening has been shown to cut the risk of a heart attack/stroke and prolong life by as much as thirty per cent among the 60s and over age group. And walking on grass, as Gulshan does every morning, has beneficial physiological effects as the Earth's surface has a negative charge and is constantly generating electrons that could neutralize free radicals, acting as antioxidants. Antioxidants are normally thought to come from food alone—a diet rich in fruits, vegetables, and other foods that provide beta-carotene, selenium, lutein, lycopene, and vitamins A, C and E helps prevent cellular damage from free radicals[56]. But earthing provides these too.

A DASH OF FORBIDDEN FOODS, NOT TOO MUCH

People who are strict disciplinarians often have higher anxiety levels. When you start taking your nutrition discipline or exercise discipline too seriously, you're building up stress which leads to inflammation and accelerated ageing. Whether you look at Ronnie, Laurence, or even Gulshan, each one of them indulges in something or the other that is not touted as 'healthy'. It could be a sugar-laden French dessert, or vodka or non-vegetarian food, but it is the quantities consumed that matter. Just two spoons, just one drink, just a bit, was something I heard each one of them say during conversations. This is a form of self-nurturing in tiny ways, every day. And these small quantities are ensuring that everything else which is healthy is on track.

Just two hundred calories of indulgence can inspire an individual to follow healthy habits like a nutritious diet, breath work, and moderate exercise more consistently daily.

And since consistency in healthy habits is what causes reduced ageing, this small indulgence is aiding that process.

When we get into a diet, and there is a severe calorie deficit, the body gets into fat storage mode. Very often, we come across women who don't eat much and exercise a lot but are unable to lose weight. I have had so many people struggling with weight gain and trying everything from crash diets to fad diets to two hours of exercise every day for one year and not losing a gram. This is because their body has been signalled into fat storage, something that humans were designed for during times of starvation. When we were hunters and gatherers in the Stone Age, a feast would be rare and fat storage was necessary for survival because starvation mode would be on at other times. However, with no dearth of food now, the body's response to starvation is the same as overindulgences—in both scenarios there is fat storage[57]. Sadly, in today's times, there is as much cellular stress created by overeating as stress created by starvation, and it puts the brakes on our ability to burn fat.

But it is easy to trick the body with modern nutritional programmes.

A cheat meal can boost the metabolism by increasing leptin, the anti-starvation hormone that sends hunger messages to the body. When your body senses a calorie deficit, leptin levels drop, prompting the metabolism to slow down and conserve energy. Throwing a tiny calorie-rich cheat meal tricks your body and brain into thinking food is plentiful and that it's okay to burn fat stored in the body. And that is why, when we see irritatingly thin people taking a couple of bites of a sinful dessert or a carbohydrate and saturated fat-rich meal, we wonder how they stay so thin. It is because they have tricked their body into believing that there is no starvation mode without even realizing this science. People with both longevity and good health are almost always doing this small amount of cheating daily. Small amounts, not too much.

STAYING IN TOUCH

The worst thing you can do is get into a lonely spot. Always remember: if you are mentally alive and fit, disease, depression, and a low quality of life will not come near you. And a large part of being mentally fit comes from staying in touch and communicating with people who relate to you.

We all were heartbroken at the news of Sushant Singh Rajput, the 34-year-old promising Indian actor, committing suicide. Reportedly, he was living alone during the pandemic lockdown. Nobody expected it, not many knew that he was on antidepressants. Isolation causes anxiety and can play havoc with the mind. And once the mind is not in control, it is unpredictable in its actions. A momentary loss of balance can cause this extreme step.

Today there are so many online options of staying in touch that it is easy to schedule your day between work, reading, exercise, and video calls with loved ones. At 81, Ronnie is doing just that. He schedules time with loved ones twice a day and even on his 81st birthday during the lockdown, he baked himself a cake and did a video call with loved ones and cut the cake before popping the champagne and saying cheers virtually.

Never allow yourself to be alone for too long, and always reach out to people you love at least once a week. Initially, you may need to push yourself to do it, but once you jot down the number of people you want to keep in touch with, scheduling them for each day of the week becomes easier and you also look forward to having these conversations on a weekly basis.

Here, I would also like to pause and give advice to people who are staying away from their ageing parents. Ageing parents can get lonely and isolated especially when they can't get out of the house much and their immune system is also low. I get so many calls from middle-aged working professionals living thousands of miles away from parents. I have put down specific tips for them to help their ageing parents cope with distance and solitude and not succumb to loneliness or depression. These are:

1. **Help them create a structure for the day** A schedule creates predictability, they will have things to look forward to. For example, on waking up, they can have herbal tea followed by deep breathing. Gently cajole them to do it every day for better immunity.

2. **On waking up, a freehand stretches routine before breakfast** You can make this schedule for them and email it. Discuss options for breakfast. They will get excited talking about food choices and look forward to the beginning of their day.

3. **After breakfast, some household work** This will help them keep busy and facilitate movement for circulation. It could be light household work, but they need to do it every day to get a sense of usefulness. A lot of old people do not have purpose in their life and that causes loneliness. Knowing that they are responsible for a particular task is important.

4. **After that they can go for a bath** A cleansing routine after you have done some work makes you feel relaxed.

5. **After this, a video call should be scheduled with you or your sibling** If it is at a specific time every day, they will look forward to it instead of feeling lonely.

6. **After the video call, they prepare lunch** After lunch, tell them it is important to lie down for at least half an hour, if not more, to give energy to the digestive system for nutrients to get absorbed. In older people, nutrient absorption is low and lying down after a meal accelerates this process, helping with immunity.

7. **When they get up, set up another video call, even if it's for five minutes** Again, the predefined time will make them look forward to it.

8. **Repeat breathing exercises** Once the call with children is done, they must repeat breathing exercises. Very important for lowering inflammation and increasing immunity to do this twice a day for older people, it also keeps their lungs and digestive system stronger.

9. **Music therapy is a must** After the video call, they should play music of their choice while they prepare dinner. Music is extremely important to reduce anxiety and create positivity. If you know the kind of music they like, create seven playlists (one for each day of the week). This will help them listen to the different kinds of music they like, and they will start looking forward to that activity as well. And it will also help them remain in a positive mood when eating food.

10. **Post-dinner video session with a loved one** After food, they should set up another video call, with either

some friends or relatives who are positive people. You can help formulate a list of people they have not been in touch with, some friends they may not have spoken with for some time, and some relatives that they were fond of but haven't been able to keep in touch with. This is a good time to catch up with people via video calls. I know a lot of older people doing this and really enjoying themselves. It also beats loneliness and even with physical distancing, they don't feel isolated.

11. **Speak to them about doing some gardening** You can easily order small pots of tulsi, curry leaves, lemongrass which they can keep in the house, tend to, and eat. When we are nurturing other living things, even if it is plants, our innate wish to live longer and positivity increases. That is why in most communities where longevity has been high, gardening has been one of the biggest drivers for older people.

I have put everything in points so that every day on the call you can check these points and help your ageing parents become disciplined in their daily structure. Once they have the structure in place and start getting used to it, they will have a purpose in life. For example, the thought process will be:

Oh God I must finish this; my son is going to call.

Oh dear, I must do this on time, I must finish my breathing exercises. I must water the plants.

This creates a purpose in life. And a purpose in life pushes us to be healthier, structured, and invest in having a strong mind.

ME TIME

What is me time? Me time is time spent with yourself; it could be enjoying your own company or doing an activity that you enjoy without feeling guilty or obligated.

While we are talking about isolation leading to depression, me time leads to self-nurturing and self-love. And both these are extremely important, not only for a healthy life but a healthy mind too. For example, Gulshan goes to the club every evening to spend time with his friends. That is his me time, and he looks forward to it. Ronnie's me time is with his peace lilies in his little garden. Laurence likes to drive down to the mountains to be with trees. I like to put on Sufi music and do gentle yoga. I know many people who like to just sit in a favourite spot in the house and read a book. Others like to listen to music. Whatever you want to do and are unable to do and keep wishing you could, as a hobby for instance, is classified as me time.

Many women struggle with this because they are either looking after kids, husband or in-laws, supervising household help, or working. They don't get a window in between to just nurture themselves with an activity that gives them joy. Which is why, more and more women are getting anxiety-related issues, depression, and hormonal imbalances including hormonal cancers. India has the largest number of depressed women[58] and the number one cancer in India is breast cancer[59]. Me time releases the anxiety you are facing on a day-to-day basis.

How do you identify if you need me time? If you are continuously exhausted, that is the first and most important sign to watch out for. According to Harvard Health Publishing, when you're exhausted, you'll shift into the amygdala, the emotional part of the brain that controls the fight or flight response, which is good against a bear attack, not so much against your child/family/work. A break ever so often reduces this fight or flight response. Always remember—when you want to nurture people around you, you cannot pour from an empty cup. If you are exhausted, crabby, and stressed, you're not going to be well-equipped to look after others, let alone yourself. Then, in a crisis, you yourself will collapse.

The benefits of me time are amazing. It empties your brain from other worries and helps you enjoy the task at hand and be in the moment. And then simultaneously, we begin to heal—inflammation levels and stress levels reduce, repair work begins, and we start to repair. The immune system responds to this winding down by becoming stronger, because the digestive system has stopped producing acids that it did in a state of chronic stress.

Consistent and structured me time helps you repair and start adopting a positive outlook towards life, hence impacting what we are always running after—a wonderful quality of life! And all you need to take out is twenty to thirty minutes of time every day for yourself. That isn't so difficult!

How to assign me time

Assign a specific time of the day Inform your family members that at this time of the day, you are unavailable to them. They may crib and disturb you, but within a week to ten days, they will start accepting it. Once you have crossed that hurdle, the other hurdle you will find is a few jibes that will come your way. Don't let it bother you. The universe is not going to change in half an hour of your not being there for your loved ones. The moment you are firm, but smiling and affectionate, about snatching away this time, slowly, the jibes will also disappear. And then a time will come when some of your family members will start imitating you. By this time, you would have already felt the benefits and they would have seen that your moods are better and your outlook towards life is more positive. That is the time to help your family members discover this wonderfully therapeutic activity.

So, what are some of the things that you can consider doing? I'm listing down what has been seen as therapeutic and is extremely easy to do and access:

1. **Go to the terrace of your building** Just sitting and watching the other buildings around is a feast for the eyes. Make sure you leave your mobile phone behind. Even if you spend fifteen minutes doing this, it will start relaxing you. The fresh air and sunlight will invigorate you and help nutrient and vitamin D absorption.

2. **Shut the door** If you have the luxury of a separate room where you can listen to music or read, tell everybody that at this time, they should not knock, enter the room or disturb you. You could also do meditation or breathing exercises without interruption at this time.

3. **Play a game** Many of us find games like Scrabble or doing the crossword therapeutic and invigorating. You may be playing on your phone, but you can switch off

all other notifications and tell your family members not
to bother you at this time.

4. **Exercise** Choose a form of exercise that you enjoy. It
could be dancing alone in a room, playing tennis against
a wall by only focusing on the activity of hitting the
ball, basketball, jogging to music, going for a walk, or
doing gentle yoga to slow meditation music. Any form
of exercise, when done alone without interruption, is
going to make you feel extremely good. It empties your
mind from interruptions and pressure and releases
endorphins, making you feel relaxed and positive.

BEING MENTALLY ACTIVE

I started my community—*RachnaRestores*—a few years ago so
that the impact of helping people stay healthy would multiply.
I alone could not achieve much impact—one person versus
many was my logic—so I instituted a professionally accredited
certification course online to help those who want to gain the
knowledge and help heal others with holistic nutrition. We
have a two hundred-plus coaches across twenty-seven countries
of all age groups. To my delight, our oldest coach is 65 years
old, who has been a schoolteacher all her life. She retired and
wanted to do something different. She was interested in the
field of health and disease reversal because her daughter was
going through a health crisis. She signed up for the course
and became a certified holistic health coach practitioner at 65
without any background in nutrition or health. And she did
not stop at helping her own daughter. She actively works with
the younger coaches, and some of them are just 22 years old,

to keep herself abreast on ways to heal people, ways to get new clients. This is true neuroplasticity.

A few days ago, she sent me this message:

> *Here in Kamshet, near Lonavala, we have a place in a senior citizen complex. I see many people suffering from varied chronic and age-related illnesses. Knowledge from your books, course notes and information from regular WhatsApp messages help me a lot. I do not interfere in their medications or what their doctors have told them. I just try to help them change their food habits and lifestyle. Walks, exercises and breathing exercises. We have yoga experts here, I do it with their help.*
>
> *I just don't want to miss out on anything.*
>
> *Warm wishes,*
> *Susmita Bagchi*

At 65 years, Susmitaji's mental agility is ensuring that she is healthy and curious and that is the biggest anti-ageing input anybody can gift themselves. Whatever age you are, challenge your brain—learn a new activity every six months. It could be a short online course, a new language, an instrument like the piano or guitar or taking professional training in singing or a form of dance. All of these will keep you mentally curious, alive, and slow down the ageing process.

Positivity

Positivity is the outcome of the mind–body connect. All the people I interviewed and those I have helped recover from chronic diseases, exhibit this positivity. It is demonstrated by the change in response to stress, gratitude, and helping others.

When you look at what Susmitaji is doing or Ronnie's excitement over lilies growing in 46°C or Laurence being peaceful about ageing well, these are signs of mental peace. When we achieve that equilibrium, positivity sets in—about the present and the future—making a person not only amiable to live with but also delightful in many ways. The antidote of positivity is negativity, which is experienced by people who are not in sync with themselves. We have already read about that lack of balance and consequent poor health.

2

Steps to Achieve the Balance

Living a nutritionally optimal life does not mean letting go of life's pleasures. People who live well and long, without disease, always indulge in a small amount of pleasure. So, what is the right balance and how can you achieve it?

The human body responds to consistency and that is what is missing with most fad diets, programmes, and treatments. People check themselves into retreats and wellness centres to get healthier. When they're done, they return to the life that gave them the health issues, bad moods, unexplained pains, and chronic fatigue in the first place. In short, most diet plans are not driven by lifestyle changes. Most diet 'plans', consultations, fads, medical or any other form of 'treatments' are reactive and focus on 'time-bound' plans to 'fix' you.

To incorporate lasting lifestyle changes that include being disease-free involves training the mind to direct the body to follow a sequential process of consistent inputs daily.

If we start following general healthy guidelines and make some changes to our lifestyle, we are going to achieve only twenty per cent of our goals. We will definitely feel better with just a few changes, but the underlying issues will not be addressed and will resurface. When you read on Dr Google that something is healthy and you incorporate it, of course it has some impact. But that impact is not long-lasting and does not do repair work.

Hence, we need to heal the body in a step-by-step process to first eliminate the causes so that symptoms can start reducing before they finally disappear.

There are things that harm you in your daily life and there are things that benefit you. Achieving the delicate balance of maintaining good health and better moods which lead to longevity consists of these four steps:

STEP 1: THE ELIMINATION PHASE

Eliminate what is harming you. It could be:

1. Smoking
2. Excessive alcohol
3. A sedentary lifestyle
4. Over-exercising
5. Foods that are harmful for specific conditions (which we will discuss in detail)
6. Overeating/junk food
7. Excess carbohydrates
8. Less sleep

Once you start understanding what is harming you, it is much easier to eliminate it so that you can focus on elements that heal you.

Why is it important to eliminate everything that can harm you in step one?

Like I gave the example of a broken bone, any other part of the body also needs sequential steps to heal. And the steps are in the form of a vertical ladder; you cannot go from step one to step four without falling off.

Step one is to eliminate anything that can hinder the process of healing. This is usually the most difficult step. However, this step yields best results. Your body will not be ready initially—that's when utilizing the mind–body connect I have spoken about comes in. This phase lasts two weeks as we take that much time to break an unhealthy habit.

During this phase, some of the elements are eliminated *permanently* (like smoking, excessive drinking or eating junk food) and others may be eliminated temporarily.

Many people come to me and say they cannot suddenly give up drinking or smoking. But I have had cases where patients have successfully quit cold turkey. While there are some benefits of moderate drinking, there is absolutely no health benefit in smoking.

How to give up smoking

Use chamomile A medicinal plant used mainly in treatment of stomach and intestinal diseases, chamomile has therapeutic properties that help heart health, reduction of type 2 diabetes symptoms, and gut repair. Since tobacco and smoking impact the entire body and can trigger a stroke or heart attack, effects of switching to chamomile are more than just reducing your urge to smoke. The damage caused by tobacco can partially get reversed.

Every time you get the urge to smoke, make yourself a cup of chamomile tea. The chamomile leaves have an effect similar to smoking. If the urge is too much, instead of drinking the tea, tear open the sachet and chew on the chamomile leaves. Do not exceed three cups a day, as chamomile induces drowsiness.

Get sage Health benefits of sage include reducing chest congestion. It acts as a natural antidepressant and mood uplifter, repressing the urge to light up a cigarette or chew tobacco. Dried sage leaves can be crushed and put into a tea concoction or chewed (half a teaspoon is more than enough at a time, twice daily). Sage supplements are also available with dosages written.

Have damiana This herb is known for creating a slight 'high' as well as increasing sexual health. For heavy smokers, sexual health is always a concern due to suppressed sperm count as a side effect of smoking. This herb also takes care of withdrawal symptoms like twitches and low moods. It is easily available as a homeopathic medicine over the counter. However, it is best to go to a homeopathic doctor and get correct dosages prescribed as per your smoking/tobacco habits.

How to give up excess alcohol

Excessive drinking has many drawbacks. The biggest one is the increased risk for oesophageal, head, neck, and many stomach cancers along with fatty liver, liver cancer, liver dysfunction, and kidney failure. However, just switching alcohol and reducing quantities has the opposite effect.

Switch from hard liquor, beer, or any other form of alcohol to red wine Two goblets, twice a week if you are a regular drinker. Each goblet is 150 ml. For people who drink hard liquor, and have not had red wine before, despite the low alcohol content in red wine, they will still experience the high they seek from excessive alcohol. At the same time, because of the presence of grapes and resveratrol, red wine is extremely anti-inflammatory. With an alcohol content of eleven to thirteen per cent, it is substantially lower than the forty per cent alcohol content of whisky, vodka, rum, etc. The quantities listed above will start reducing cravings and inflammation related to excessive hard liquor. Some may face acidity with red wine; this is indicative of poor gut.

Also remember—even if you drink once a week or once a month, but you go overboard with the hard liquor, it still makes you a heavy drinker. This is because when you binge drink, you're overloading your body and your liver. Whether you do it once a week or once a month, it is better to be consistent with lower quantities of alcohol. Red wine will also help you wean off cravings and withdrawal symptoms while protecting your organs if consumed in the quantities written above. During the elimination phase, you can have listed quantities if you get cravings.

For non-drinkers, please don't start drinking red wine in this phase, though it is fine to have it once you are in the last phase, which is the lifestyle phase.

What foods to give up and why

Wheat, white flour, gluten Whether you are trying to prevent or manage/reverse the disease, the way wheat is produced is the issue. We have all developed gluten intolerances only because we are getting GMO wheat in most parts of the world except parts of Europe. And the way we make bread also does not break down gluten. Gluten is a protein found in wheat which cannot be absorbed by the small intestines and stops other nutrients from being absorbed. Even though gluten is an important nutrient and wheat itself has a lot of fibre, minerals and proteins, most people who get off gluten start feeling better. Increasingly, research is showing that the way modern-day wheat is produced is impairing the gut. A child's intake of gluten at eighteen months is associated with a forty-six per cent increased risk of developing type 1 diabetes for each extra ten grams of gluten consumed[60]. Apart from hindering absorption of nutrients, it also increases sugar spikes, causes hormonal fluctuations, and skin issues. Wheat in any form can also trigger a harmful immune response in immunocompromised people, and most people I know have low immunity in any case if they're stressed out.

So if you are stressed out, or trying to prevent, manage, or reverse any inflammatory condition like heart disease, cholesterol, blockages, type 2 diabetes, unexplained pains, weight gain, and hormonal issues like PCOS or thyroid, the first step is to eliminate gluten. This will ensure that your gut will not react, it will be easier to pacify; and repair of gut is the purpose of healing. Once the gut is repaired, its absorption of nutrients, elimination of waste and transfer of nutrients to the rest of the body becomes more efficient, leading to lower inflammation and higher immunity.

Most of you will be able to come back to incorporating gluten into your diet occasionally. Even for those who do not have gluten intolerance or coeliac disease, it is advisable to eliminate all forms of gluten which include wheat, white flour, rye, and semolina, at this stage.

Milk and milk products As an animal protein, milk is inflammatory and contains sugar, in the form of lactose. Any form of sugar or inflammatory foods at this stage will hinder the journey of healing because we are trying to reduce inflammation levels and if we include anything that increases them, we are going one step forward and two steps backwards. I have written about this in my other books as well. Milk has been linked to triggering not only inflammation[61] but heart disease[62], type 2 diabetes, and certain types of hormonal cancers. Milk causes mucous in the body, and mucous feeds bad cells.

Animal protein All forms of animal proteins at this stage should be eliminated because of their inherent inflammatory nature. At a later stage, for animal protein lovers, organic eggs and oily fish will be brought back, so don't despair. In almost all studies done on animal protein, especially red meat, processed meat has been linked to lifestyle diseases and cancer. Studies show there is no inflammation with organic and grass-fed meats but at this stage, even those should be avoided. We are trying to expel the toxins with the elimination phase, anything difficult to digest is going to hinder that.

Lentils and pulses Yes, I hear you saying, why? Why? Because lentils and pulses are acidic in nature and anything acidic increases inflammation and hinders the journey of gut repair. Once your healing is complete, and to maintain stability, you can add these foods back in small parts. The exceptions are people recovering from cancer, those who have gout, bone pain or autoimmune condition. For them, lentils and pulses should be permanently eliminated.

Sugar Processed sugar and even any form of healthy sugar in large quantities is prohibited at this stage. I know a lot of people who take pride in being healthy and will eat large quantities of quinoa cake (gluten-free) with date syrup (natural sugar). If you're having a two-inch slice, it's understandable. However, when you overload the body with any sugar, whether it is natural sugar from fruits, raw honey or jaggery, or table sugar, the body experiences a sugar rush which increases inflammation. With the exception of raw organic honey and two dates, twice a week (optional). Raw honey has natural probiotics and minerals to repair the gut and should be taken in small quantities, and a few dates, two to three times a week, are good for your thyroid. All the other so-called healthy sugars, including dark chocolate, are not allowed because they will irritate the gut.

TIPS TO MAKE YOUR DETOX SUCCESSFUL

Here are some tips to help you achieve the success that you are seeking:

Read through the plan listed and stock up Any plan will fail if you have not prepared in advance. Plan your week so that you can eat healthy and do not deviate and reach for other options because you did not plan well. Stock up on vegetables, fruits, and carbohydrates listed so that there is never any excuse of not having them available at the time you need them.

This plan is about specifics You cannot replace one fruit with another, one carbohydrate with another, one salad item with another, one oil with another. This phase is about detoxing you. All ingredients listed work in combination with each other, so don't change things around just because you read somewhere, or someone told you something else is healthy for you. Make your life easier—if it is not written, don't do it. If it is written, follow it. My plans are scientifically tested!

Purchase a weighing scale Take your weight reading every morning after going to the bathroom. This will help you stay on track in terms of understanding toxins release. You will notice that the days you ate a late dinner, had less water, and changed the combinations a bit, you will not lose weight. However, every single day that you follow the plan, you will lose weight even if it is fifty grams. Weight is an indicator at this stage of toxins being expelled.

Always keep a bottle of water with you Staying hydrated is half the battle won. If you keep sipping water through the day, your true hunger will emerge versus the hunger that emerges when we are dehydrated. Drinking water also increases your BMR, releases toxins, clears up your skin, and lowers blood pressure. Water helps transport oxygen and nutrients critical to the brain cells and you will always stay calm if you are hydrated. When you are calm, good decision-making will help you stay on track with your plan.

Not infused water, not lemon water, just pure and simple water. It is the most powerful tool for a healthy life.

Here's what your fifteen-day detox plan looks:

THE 15-DAY DETOX

Day 1 to 7

On waking up Go to the bathroom, come out and record your weight and vital statistics. A lot of people end up losing as much as one to three kilos during this period and it will be a big win if you lose even one kilo! Recording your weight at the start and end of the plan along with measurements will help you understand the amount you have achieved in these fifteen days in expelling toxins.

Within 30 minutes of waking up 200 ml water, one cup pure green tea (no flavours), preferably loose tea leaves and not sachets. You can add crushed tulsi leaves. With five raw almonds, not roasted, not soaked.

Do deep breathing exercise Five counts Sheetali, five minutes Anulom Vilom, five counts Bhramari, as directed on p. 76-80.

After breathing exercises: breakfast Choose any three from these seven fruits: one apple, ten medium-sized pieces of papaya, five red or black grapes, half pomegranate, two slices pineapple, five berries of any kind. Make a fruit bowl. Add ten almonds and ten pistachios. Eat slowly. Followed by one cup of green tea.

Two hours later (snack) 200 ml water, one bowl (ten to eleven pieces) roasted fox nuts (makhanas) or five pistachios if fox nuts are not available. Followed by one cup green tea.

Lunch (1.30-2 p.m.) Six to seven tablespoons of boiled brown rice (cooked quantity), ten tablespoons of cooked vegetables.

Cook the vegetables lightly with less oil. You must add a pinch of turmeric, a pinch of black pepper. You can also season with whole spices, herbs, onions, garlic, ginger, green or red chillies (all optional). Do not use packet masalas as they have toxins, you can use whole spices. All green vegetables are fine, use variety, eat local, rotate vegetables, no potatoes, sweet potatoes (at this stage only).

When vegetables are on your plate, pour four (yes four, do not reduce) tablespoons of extra virgin olive oil over them. Extra virgin olive oil should be in a glass bottle and have 'cold pressed' or 'cold extracted' or 'first pressed' written somewhere on the bottle.

After lunch Sit for thirty minutes without your phone and laptop. Preferably lie down on the left side if you can. Your digestive system needs energy to absorb nutrients and send them to various parts of the body. Any movement is going to dissipate the energy source.

3.30 p.m. Two glasses of water (200 ml each), sipped slowly, one cup green tea.

4.30 p.m. Five minutes of Anulom Vilom, done in an unhurried manner, with music.

Evening time (5–5.30 p.m.) One cup green tea, one tablespoon each of chia and pumpkin seeds, raw, not roasted. Add sea/pink salt for taste. Do not use table salt for anything.

6 p.m. Two glasses of water (200 ml each), sipped slowly.

6.45 p.m. Soup

One cup soup Any two fresh veggies per day in soup, rotate these. Combinations can be—carrot-doodhi (bottle gourd), cabbage-peas, French beans-carrots, fenugreek leaves-coriander/parsley, cauliflower-tori, broccoli-spinach. Wash well, chop, add half cup water, boil in pressure cooker, cool down (don't touch it for forty-five minutes), open, blend into a smooth paste, add herbs and sea salt. If you don't get the combinations listed, you can use any two vegetables but avoid vegetables with seeds like tomatoes, brinjal, capsicum, bell peppers. Ladies finger or okra is fine.

Dinner (7 p.m.) Five tablespoons boiled brown rice, cooled, tossed into a salad of finely chopped Romaine lettuce, onions and cucumber. If not available, use 'salad leaves' which are easily available with any vegetable vendor or freshly-chopped coriander/parsley/celery as per availability. Add green chillies (optional), sea/pink salt to taste, black pepper, herbs (optional), fresh coriander/parsley (if you get lettuce). Add three tablespoons of extra virgin olive oil (mandatory). Toss together and enjoy.

10 p.m. One cup chamomile tea (do not skip, even if you are a non-smoker).

10.30 p.m. Lights out. It is important that you follow this schedule of getting into bed early to pacify your cortisol levels and accelerate the detoxification process.

No exercise for seven days. Not even walks. No matter what. Remember at this stage if you exercise, you are going to stop the energy from going to your gut to accelerate the detoxification process. So, don't listen to anybody else; this process only works if energy to the gut is uninterrupted.

Day 8 to 15

In week two, food inclusions are small but significant, so please read carefully; however, exercise is added.

On waking up Go to the bathroom, come out and record the following, this will be required to monitor your progress:

Weight
Chest/bust
Waist
Hip
Upper thigh measurements

If you have followed the first seven days of the plan exactly as written without deviations in food, timings, breathing exercises, combinations, water intake and sleep, you would have lost a little bit of weight and inches as well. This is an indicator of your body responding to consistency. If the consistent input has been missing, you can either restart or ensure that now onwards consistency is not missing, otherwise it will not positively impact your body in becoming disease-free.

Within 30 minutes of waking up 200 ml water, one cup pure green tea (no flavours), preferably loose tea leaves and not sachets. Ten raw almonds, not roasted, not soaked.

After green tea and almonds Warm-up exercises as given below:

Warm-up exercise before walk/jog
For instructions, see p. 128

1

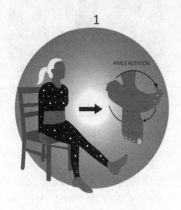

2

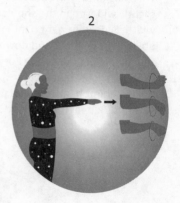

3

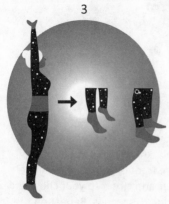

4

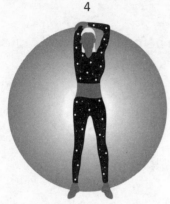

5

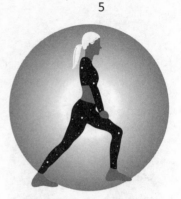

Triceps: Stand with your feet slightly wider than the shoulder width. Slide your right hand up, over your head, and down the middle of your spine. Push gently on your right elbow with your left hand, hold for 10 seconds. Repeat on other side. Do thrice.

Hamstrings: Stand with your left leg in front of the right. Bend your right knee and tilt your hips as you rest weight on your upper right thigh. Your front leg should be straight, toes pointing up. Hold for 10 seconds. Repeat on the other leg. Do thrice.

6

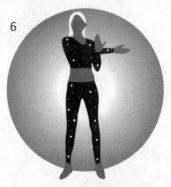

Shoulders: Stand tall, your feet slightly wider than the shoulder width, with your knees slightly bent. Place your right arm across the front of your chest, parallel to the ground. Bring your arm closer to your chest and your left forearm. Hold for 10 seconds. Repeat on the other side. Do thrice.

After warm-up exercises Twenty minutes moderate-paced walk inside the house or compound on an even surface. *Do not walk fast or slow*, do not stop in between to check something or talk to somebody.

After walk Breathing exercises (see p. 76-80) as listed below, these are mandatory, do not skip them.

1. Five minutes Sheetali.
2. Ten minutes Anulom Vilom.
3. Five counts Bhramari.

Breakfast Choose any three from these seven in the quantities listed: one apple, ten medium-sized pieces of papaya, five red or black grapes, half pomegranate, two slices pineapple, five berries of any kind. Make a fruit bowl. Add ten almonds and ten pistachios. Eat slowly. Followed by one cup green tea.

Two hours later 200 ml water. Snack options (as per availability):

1. One cup green tea, half mashed avocado, add sea salt as per taste, with two to three Rice Crackers (see p. 212).
2. One bowl (ten to eleven pieces) roasted fox nuts (makhanas).
3. Ten pistachios.

Followed by one cup green tea.

Lunch options, as per availability (1.30-2 p.m.)

1. Two Rice Cutlets (see p. 225), ten tablespoons of cooked vegetables.

2. Two Quinoa Methi Tikki (see p. 228), ten tablespoons of cooked vegetables.
3. Only on Sunday afternoon (treat): Mackerel Biryani (see p. 226).

Cook vegetables lightly with less or no oil. You can season with whole spices, herbs, onions, garlic, ginger, green or red chillies. Do not use packet masalas. All green vegetables are fine, no potatoes or sweet potatoes. When the vegetables are on your plate, pour four tablespoons of extra virgin olive oil on the vegetables.

After lunch Close your eyes and lie down, preferably on your left side.

3.30 p.m. Two glasses of water (200 ml each).

4.30 p.m. Fifteen minutes Anulom Vilom only, to music.

Evening time (5–5.30 p.m.) One green tea with (as per taste/availability):

1. Two pieces of Quinoa Cake (see p. 213).
2. One tablespoon each of chia and pumpkin seeds, raw, not roasted, two tablespoons puffed rice. Toss together, add chopped onions, fresh coriander. Add sea/pink salt for taste. Do not use table salt for anything.

6.30 p.m. Two glasses of water. Ten minutes moderate-paced walk. Do not exceed.

Dinner (7 p.m.) 50g boiled quinoa, cooled, tossed into salad made of chopped lettuce/salad/coriander/parsley/celery, onions, cucumber.

For salad dressing Three tablespoons of extra virgin olive oil, five crushed walnuts (all three mandatory), one tablespoon raw honey, one teaspoon mustard (both optional, for taste only). Toss together and enjoy. Do not exceed quantities.

10 p.m. One cup chamomile tea.

10.30 p.m. Lights out (it is important that you follow this schedule of getting into bed early to pacify your cortisol levels to hasten detoxification process). In the initial few days if you are not used to sleeping at this time, you will toss and turn for a bit but after a few days, your body will adjust.

No other exercise except what is listed. *No matter what.* Remember, at this stage if you exercise more, you are going to stop the energy from going to your gut to accelerate the detoxification process.

Step 2: The repair phase

By this time, your cravings for junk food, smoking, tobacco and excessive alcohol should have died down. Some discomfort in the form of acidity, bloating and headaches can be experienced by people with a compromised gut, hormonal issues, and severe dependencies on higher carbohydrates, smoking, and alcohol.

Now, you are ready to incorporate everything that will repair you.

Once you have eliminated what can harm and hinder your journey of healing, even if some foods are only temporarily cut out, many people start feeling fresher and experience better moods. Waking up is easier and sleep patterns have started to set in. Those aiming for weight loss would have lost a little more weight by now.

Now, you must incorporate a healing lifestyle so that repair work can begin and eventually stabilize the gut and body. This means that the correct balance of anti-inflammatory nutrients, exercise schedule and breathing techniques must be part of this repairing process. This phase lasts *three weeks*.

We are moving towards more options for meals, snacks. Please make sure you stick to only the options mentioned and exercises given are followed on specified days. Swapping ingredients or exercises is not an option if you want the right output.

Day 16 to 37

On waking up Go to the bathroom, come out and record the following to monitor your progress:

Weight
Chest/bust
Waist
Hip
Upper thigh measurements

Within thirty minutes of waking up 200 ml water, one cup pure green tea (no flavours), preferably green tea leaves and not sachets. Ten raw almonds, not roasted, not soaked.

Warm-up exercises as given earlier, followed by:

Monday, Wednesday, Friday Forty minutes moderate-paced walk on an even surface like home, compound, or park. Do not walk fast or slow, do not stop in between to check something or talk to somebody.

Tuesday, Thursday, Saturday After warm-up, climb down five flights of stairs and climb back up. Do it slowly, do not run up or down as this can cause you to fall or put pressure on your heart. Even if you do not have a history of heart disease, please adhere to this warning very carefully. Climb down very slowly and climb up even more slowly taking at least thirty to forty minutes to complete the entire five storeys, up and down combined. Any rushing, fast exercise or running is going to upset the plan and can endanger your heart, muscles, and lead to injury.

Do not skip this exercise, do it as written, slowly, without jerky movements, for best results. Do not do this if you have a knee problem. For those with knee problems, a twenty-five-minute walk is enough.

After exercise Breathing exercises (see p. 76-80) as listed below, these are mandatory; do not skip them.

1. Five minutes Sheetali.
2. Ten minutes Anulom Vilom.
3. Ten counts Bhramari.

After breathing exercises (breakfast options to rotate):

1. Fruit Smoothie (see p. 215).
2. Super Seeds Fruit and Nut Smoothie (see p. 232).

Two hours later 200 ml water. Ten almonds and ten pistachios. Followed by one cup green tea.

Lunch (1.30–2 p.m.)

Monday, Wednesday, Friday One Salted Pancake/Cheela/Uttapam (see p. 208). Have with two different vegetables.

You must add a pinch of turmeric, a pinch of black pepper. Cook vegetables lightly with less or no oil. You can season with whole spices, herbs, onions, garlic, ginger, green or red chillies. Do not use packet masalas. All green vegetables are fine, no potatoes. When vegetables are on your plate, pour three tablespoons of extra virgin olive oil (combined) on all the vegetables. Keep a small bottle of extra virgin olive oil in your office so that you can pour it fresh.

Tuesday, Thursday, Saturday One Roti/Salted Pancake (see p. 208). With two vegetables. Cooking and seasoning instructions as given above.

Sunday Zoodles with a Cashew Moringa Pesto (see p. 233).

After lunch Sit for thirty minutes without phone and laptop and close your eyes. Try and lie down, preferably on your left side.

3 p.m. Two glasses of water (200 ml each).

Evening time (5–5.30 p.m.) options:

1. Sweet potato chaat: Boil or roast, peel and chop some fresh greens/onions. Sprinkle sea salt, crack some black pepper, add a tablespoon of yoghurt or extra virgin olive oil, and toss together. A perfect, nourishing summer snack!

2. Fruit chaat: Choose between these three fruits in the quantities listed: one apple, ten medium-sized pieces of papaya, five red or black grapes, half pomegranate, and two slices pineapple. Choose any three and make a fruit bowl. Add chaat masala, other flavours as per taste. Eat slowly. Followed by one cup green tea.

3. Apple and Fig Cobbler (see p. 230).

6.30 p.m. Twenty minutes of moderate-paced walk around the office, home, or compound. Do not walk fast or slow, do not stop in between to check something or talk to somebody. Followed by two glasses of water, one cup green tea.

Dinner (7 p.m.) options:

1. Rainbow Buddha Bowl (see p. 231).
2. Moong sprouts salad 50 g (five tablespoons) sprouted moong (see p. 216 for how to sprout moong), tossed into salad (finely chopped) of Romaine lettuce. If not available, use 'salad leaves' which are easily available with any vegetable vendor or fresh chopped coriander/ parsley/celery as per availability, add cucumber, onion, green chillies (optional), sea/pink salt to taste, black pepper, herbs (optional), fresh coriander/parsley (if you get lettuce). Add three tablespoons of extra virgin olive oil (mandatory). Toss together and enjoy.
3. Hundred grams fish (no Basa) grilled/pan-fry in less oil, tossed into salad of finely chopped romaine lettuce. If not available, use 'salad leaves'. Follow seasoning instructions given above.
4. Kale and Quinoa Salad with Avocado (see p. 219).
5. Tofu Salad (see p. 224).
6. Two organic eggs boiled and tossed into a salad of finely chopped romaine lettuce. If not available, use 'salad leaves'. Follow seasoning instructions from Moong sprouts salad (above).

For salad dressing Three tablespoons of extra virgin olive oil, two tablespoons yoghurt (both mandatory), one tablespoon honey, one teaspoon mustard (optional). Toss together and enjoy. Do not exceed yoghurt quantities.

10 p.m. One cup chamomile tea.

10.30 p.m. Lights out. It is important that you follow this schedule of getting into bed early to pacify your cortisol levels to increase the detoxification process and weight loss.

No other exercise except what is listed. *No matter what.*

Step 3: The stabilization phase

In this phase, the continuity of balance needs to be consistent for the immune system to stabilize and inflammation levels to reduce.

How is this different from step two? In step two, when you are introducing only healing elements and exercise, you will face a certain amount of discomfort. If you have a compromised gut, you will have experienced bloating, acidity, and constipation. If you ate more carbohydrates earlier which induce addictiveness—and these could be wheat, white flour, corn, excess food in terms of the number of calories you consume, junk foods, excess alcohol, smoking, sedentary lifestyle—you will face headaches because there will be withdrawal symptoms or constipation which also causes headaches. Hence, your ability to follow through with phase 2 will be mired in certain difficulties which will get streamlined by the time you reach phase 3.

In phase 3, consistency of input will be more regular, higher, and structured because you will begin to enjoy the benefits of the detox in the form of freshness, weight loss, higher energy, better sleep, and a much more efficient digestive system. That stability will be achieved in this phase and for those of you who have medical conditions that have shown up in the reports, it is during this phase that your reports will start getting back in range (if followed as prescribed). Cholesterol levels will come down, triglycerides will reduce, high blood pressure and sugar levels will reduce, and inflammation levels of CRP and ESR—if they have been consistently high—will start reducing. This phase lasts six weeks.

By this time, you would have lost a reasonable amount of bloating and three to four kilos minimum of weight loss as well if you did everything as prescribed. Many people lose more than this.

Now we are moving towards the last two weeks to finally cement your detox and healing journey. Please make sure you stick to only the options written. Also, please make sure that the exercises given are followed as per specified days.

Day 37 to 79

On waking up Go to the bathroom, come out and record these before starting, this will be required to monitor your progress:

Weight
Chest/Bust
Waist
Hip
Upper Thigh measurements

Within thirty minutes of waking up 200 ml water, one cup pure green tea (no flavours), preferably green tea leaves and not sachets. Ten almonds, raw, not roasted, not soaked.

Monday, Wednesday, Friday Warm-up exercises as given earlier, followed by forty minutes moderate-paced walk on an even surface at home, in the compound or park. Do not walk fast or slow, do not stop in between to check something or talk to somebody.

Tuesday, Thursday, Saturday Yoga exercises as per schedule given on p. 128.

After exercise Twenty-five minutes breathing exercises as given earlier (mandatory, cannot skip).

After breathing exercises (breakfast)

Monday, Wednesday, Friday Medium-sized (six to seven tablespoons) bowl of Oats Upma (see p. 209).

Tuesday, Thursday, Saturday Omelette Pizza (see p. 222).

Two hours later 200 ml water. Ten almonds and ten pistachios. Followed by one cup green tea.

Lunch (1.30–2 p.m.) Fruit and seeds platter. Since you have had a reasonably heavy breakfast followed by nuts for snack, a light fruit lunch will help you stay detoxed and continue the weight loss. Choose any three from these fruits in the quantities listed: Half apple OR five red grapes OR black grapes OR half pomegranate OR five strawberries OR five blueberries OR one slice pineapple. And make a fruit bowl. Add one tablespoon each of sunflower, pumpkin, and chia seeds. Add chaat masala, other flavours as per taste. Eat slowly.

3.30 p.m. Two glasses of water (200 ml each).

Evening time (5–5.30 p.m.) Choose from these options:

1. Murmura (puffed rice) Chaat with Nuts (see p. 215).
2. Coffee with Fenugreek Seeds and Palm Jaggery (see p. 222).
3. One slice Savoury Italian-style Muffins (see p. 229).

Followed by one cup green tea. Can also choose from previous snacks.

6.30 p.m. Twenty minutes of moderate-paced walk around the office, home, or compound. Do not walk fast or slow, do not stop in between to check something or talk to somebody. Followed by two glasses of water, one cup green tea.

Dinner (7 p.m.)

Monday, Wednesday, Friday (for vegetarians) Moong sprouts salad 50 g (see p. 179)

Monday, Wednesday, Friday (for non-vegetarians) Two boiled organic eggs tossed into salad of Romaine lettuce. If not available, use 'salad leaves'. Follow seasoning instructions from Moong sprouts salad (see p. 179).

For salad dressing: Three tablespoons of extra virgin olive oil, two tablespoons yoghurt (both mandatory), one tablespoon honey, one teaspoon mustard (optional). Toss together and enjoy. Do not exceed yoghurt quantities.

Tuesday, Thursday, Saturday (for vegetarians) Pumpkin Soup (see p. 221). Ten almonds, five crushed walnuts and ten pistachios tossed into salad of Romaine lettuce. If not available, use 'salad leaves'. Follow seasoning instructions from Moong sprouts salad (see p. 179).

Tuesday, Thursday, Saturday (for non-vegetarians; non-vegetarians who want to eat vegetarian food some days can choose from the vegetarian options on those days) Grilled Coriander Fish (see p. 234), no Basa, to be had with salad of Romaine lettuce. If not available, use 'salad leaves'. Follow seasoning instructions from Moong sprouts salad (see p. 179).

9 p.m. One tablespoon Dairy-free Fruit Ice Cream (see p. 223).

10 p.m. One cup chamomile tea.

10.30 p.m. Lights out (It is important that you follow this schedule of getting into bed early to pacify your cortisol levels to increase the detoxification process and weight loss).

No other exercise except what is listed. *No matter what.*

STAGE 4: THE LIFESTYLE PHASE

You have incorporated healthy habits and learnt to enjoy them because you have reaped the benefits of higher energy levels, better sleep and, in many cases, disease reversal signs if you have had high cholesterol, type 2 diabetes, hypertension, hormonal fluctuations, and even severe anxiety. Now is the time to adapt them into your daily life. How do you do that without thinking of being in a restrictive environment inside your head? You must start thinking *ingredients*.

Ingredients versus recipes. This will help you create your own healthy universe on your plate.

I am listing below golden rules for having an optimum lifestyle where you can prevent future health issues after you have been through the stages of healing. Read on so you can incorporate these practices in your daily lifestyle and stay healthy for years to come.

Your past life no longer controls you To continue your journey of expelling toxins and bloating on a daily basis rather than going on fad diets, as well as making sure that your hormones are pacified (for women), you need to have carbohydrates in smaller quantities, and choose what's good for you. Wheat, white flour is *not* good and will mess up your gut. Many of you (men, not women with hormonal issues) can reintroduce wheat in small quantities to your diet but do keep it to small quantities so that the gut stays clean and healthy. Apart from wheat, you can have so many other carbohydrates. These are all kinds of rice (white, brown, red, blue), millets of all kinds (bajra, jowar, ragi), and other protein-rich carbohydrates like amaranth, quinoa, and oats.

If you have compromised digestion, anxiety, and headaches, and you may have that if your hormones are fluctuating, always stick to cooked white rice, without draining the water. *White rice is a great prebiotic and will pacify your gut.* Don't worry, you will not gain weight with boiled white rice as long as your quantities are moderate. The other food that will mess up your hormones is paneer/cottage cheese. I'm emphasizing this for vegetarians because they often compensate their protein intake with milk or paneer. Your protein choices can consist of light lentils like moong and masoor and a handful of nuts. Twice a week, take a few tablespoons of yoghurt and very small quantities of cheese like cheddar or feta. Why cheese is allowed and not paneer is because one tends to eat paneer like a vegetable. And this is when, in high quantities, paneer becomes unhealthy—it messes up your hormones and causes accumulation of belly fat. If you can eat your paneer as you would cheese—not more than 15g just twice a week—it is absolutely fine to have paneer.

Your vegetables can save you In every meal, we eat cooked vegetables (in the form of sabzi for Indians) and these vegetables, when cooked till soft on a high flame, lose their protective phytonutrient qualities that protect our heart, body, mind, and hormones. Hence, you should keep veggies crunchy and have raw salad along with every meal. Even more so if your sugar levels are high and you are overweight.

A good combination in every meal, whether it is breakfast, lunch or dinner, is to have half your meal comprise cooked food and the other half consisting of raw salads like cucumber, lettuce, carrots, onions, beetroot, and so on. Choose from seasonal varieties but have them raw and pour extra virgin olive oil on them. This not only ensures that we get the anti-cancer antioxidants present in these raw salads, the combination of salad and extra virgin olive oil pacifies the brain, lowers stress levels, and flushes out the bad fat from our body. It also ensures that our food intake is less, thereby reducing calories consumed. When we start eating less, we start to see our hormone levels getting balanced out and our moods get better. You will also see a rise in your haemoglobin level if you have raw salads like romaine lettuce, baby spinach, other leafy greens tossed with lightly cooked broccoli or French beans, cucumber, and olive oil, twice a day.

Always remember this golden rule if you want to stay healthy and have an energetic life—forty per cent of your plate needs to have salads and the other forty per cent needs to have cooked items like lentils, vegetables, roti made from gluten-free flour or rice. You will automatically start feeling lighter and healthier. The twenty per cent that remains should be empty. And no second helpings!

The fat in your food is a mood swinger It is raw, unsaturated fats, combined with salads and green vegetables, that consistently reduce anxiety levels and inflammation. I cannot emphasize this enough; I have personally seen this work for me as well as many men and women I have treated. I have even treated chronic anxiety and depression patients with this combination of food with amazing results and have gotten them off antidepressants. Unsaturated fats like extra virgin olive oil, virgin flaxseed oil and fish oil have extremely heart protective and hormone balancing properties[63]. Avoid coconut oil, even if it is virgin coconut oil, because it is saturated fat that will increase your bad fat levels.

I have had many people come to me with very high triglyceride levels, increased weight, and high cholesterol because they read somewhere that it is healthy to have virgin coconut oil. Please stay away from saturated fat in any form including butter, ghee, coconut milk, animal milk (cow, buffalo) and of course, coconut oil if you want to stay lean and have high energy without a bad lipid profile.

A thumb rule to have your good fats in the right quantities is to have two to three tablespoons of extra virgin olive oil in your salad at every meal. Never cook with extra virgin olive oil or flaxseed oil as they lose their anti-inflammatory properties when you heat them. You can use rice bran oil for cooking as it is healthy.

For those who don't have health issues, one tablespoon of saturated fat like butter/ghee/coconut oil three times a week is good but for anybody else who already has even a mild inflammatory condition or hormonal fluctuations, stay away from saturated fat. Of course, for children under ten, butter and ghee are great for brain development and should be given liberally.

Timing is key There are so many conversations and posts around intermittent fasting benefits. If you finish eating by 7 p.m. and are not eating anything before 11 a.m. the next day (as written in my plan as well), you are practising intermittent fasting daily! This is because you are going without any food for sixteen hours. Giving your stomach and digestive system a break with this kind of a gap is required mostly every day. It has to be a lifestyle change, not a fad diet you try before going back to eating late dinners and feeling sluggish in the morning.

On most days, try to finish dinner by 7 p.m. An early dinner plays a significant role in reducing stubborn belly fat. You wake up fresh in the morning to greet your day with a happy tummy as your food would have been digested well. If you have to go out for a party, eat and go. At the party, you can nibble on one or two pieces of safe snacks like fish, a handful of nuts (please be mindful of quantities), or salad. And yes, it is safe to have one or two glasses of red wine at a party once or twice a week. No other alcohol is as healthy, not even white wine.

Your plate is your window to good health Visually, half your plate should be raw foods and vegetables. This means half your plate should be a cooked vegetable and salad, one-fourth should be a protein and one-fourth a permitted carbohydrate. If you have three meals that contain these ingredients in the quantities listed, you will never gain weight or be low on energy, or haemoglobin.

All proteins are not created equal You need protein to ensure muscle mass does not decline and energy remains high. Best proteins are nuts and seeds, organic eggs and occasionally, oily fish like salmon, mackerel, anchovies, herring, and trout. Don't go for cheaper varieties of fish like basa and sole as these are nutritionally low and often adulterated.

Food must be earned You should eat when you have burnt enough calories to earn your food. This is very different from doing normal activities like going to the bathroom, running after your child, walking around the office, cooking for your family, or going to the market. I know you get tired doing these things, but the reason for that is you're not getting adequate nutrition. Once your nutrition levels are as listed earlier, your energy levels will increase with your day-to-day chores. When that happens, you should start a proper exercise routine that will help further increase them and ensure you stay fresh and lean.

While I have listed some exercises, you can always add to or continue these. The best heart-protective and hormone-pacifying exercises are moderate walking for forty-five to sixty minutes three days a week and the yoga schedule (see p. 128) given on the other three days (rest on the seventh day).

Exercise cannot be limited to one hour every day Only doing exercises at specific times of the day isn't going to keep your circulation going all through the day. If you are sitting all day and suddenly get up and exercise for an hour, your circulation will only move for that one hour. Circulation is important for nutrients to reach the body parts that need it, for the digestive system to expel toxins, for metabolic rate to be high, and for inflammation levels to remain low.

Getting up every ninety minutes from your desk/chair/bed does this trick. Stretch, go and get yourself a glass of water (instead of relying on any help), pour yourself some green tea (get those antioxidants going!) and come back to your desk for the next ninety minutes. The entire process of kick-starting your circulation with movement and hydration (water increases circulation) takes under five minutes. And look at the benefits it can have in terms of reducing the risk of all the health issues

I have listed above. The human body is made for movement, so move it!

Drink water the right way, every day Water is required to carry nutrients to various parts of the body, for circulation, to reduce blood pressure and inflammation levels, to release toxins, hydrate brain cells (which need more hydration than the other body parts), and for pretty much everything we do. We are, after all, made of seventy per cent water. So how do we clock the water in our lives without diluting the nutrients in the body?

Just like the thumb rules for body movement to increase circulation, the thumb rule for drinking water is to have some every ninety minutes of waking time. One glass of water every ninety minutes of waking time is far better than drinking larger quantities of water in one go and burdening your urinary bladder. People who drink less water are more forgetful and get frequent headaches because the brain cells need hydration on a consistent basis.

Eat twenty per cent less than your appetite We all have an anti-ageing gene called SIRT1 that gets activated by the simple function of eating less than our appetite. Now that you are on the path of continued good health, eating twenty per cent less will continue to reduce your process of ageing whether it is your organs or your physical appearance. Hence, your inflammation levels will remain low and your disease activity will be low as well, reducing your biological age. You may be forty-five years old, but you will begin to look younger and fresher. In whichever part of the world people follow this principle of restrictive eating, the population has benefitted. Look at the portion sizes of the Japanese and French and the number of veggies and raw items in the Mediterranean diet (which automatically reduce calories). While the traditional Japanese diet and way of life has proven to be the healthiest in reducing disease activity to less than three per cent, the French women paradox of eating butter, cheese, and wheat and still staying slim has bothered some scientists. But the clue lies in the quantities the French eat, and the amount they walk. The time the human body takes to digest the food and burn these calories plays an important role in eating less. When you are eating less, your digestive system is not overwhelmed, and it is functioning more efficiently to not only absorb the nutrients but also burn the calories and expel toxins.

It is difficult for people used to large quantities to shift to smaller portion sizes. No problem, you can concentrate more on vegetables and decreased quantities of carbohydrates and proteins. This will immediately decrease the number of calories. *Remember: our stomach is a little elastic bag, put in more, it expands; put in less, it shrinks. Making it shrink is easier than you think.*

TRAVEL AND EATING OUT TIPS

Living a good life is all about planning well so you can stick to a healthy lifestyle, enjoy yourself and be disease-free. When you stick to your health goals, you will realize you are a happier person and if you are a happier person, you spread this happiness to your loved ones. Your high energy also enables you to look after them much better than earlier.

Why you need a travel schedule

Why is it important to stick to a healthy living programme during your travel? If you are on holiday, you deserve a break, right? Wrong. You are on that holiday because you want to *enjoy* the holiday. The key word here is enjoy. Reverting to junk eating or foods that didn't work for you will bring back the same problems. Going berserk on a holiday is most likely going to ruin your holiday because you will have low energy, no happy tummy, and missed sunrises because you will not have the freshness to absorb the new place and get rejuvenated. Whether it is a holiday or weekend, we forget that the purpose of the holiday is to rejuvenate us, and the weekend is meant to repair us from the week's stress and irregular hours. If we remember the *purpose*, it is easy for us to not only stick to our heavy schedule, but also plan so much better.

The right nutrient balance that enhances everyday joy needs to be cherished and preserved more than **any** *wealth in the world.*

Travel schedule

On waking up (in your hotel room) Have ten almonds, one green tea (available at most hotels but ideally you should be carrying your nuts and green tea sachets). Do the basic stretches in yoga as given in phase two. It is easy to do them in the hotel room as it will only take ten minutes. This will make you feel energetic because of the circulation and joint opening and you'll be fresh to enjoy the day.

Breakfast Have fruits first. Papaya/red/black grapes/apple (whatever's available) with two eggs cooked any way you like. If you don't eat eggs, replace with ten almonds and ten pistachios or gluten-free pancakes/dishes.

Lunch/dinner A large soup-bowl size of stir-fry veggies, five to seven tablespoons of steamed white or brown rice (yes, white rice is absolutely fine if the quantities are moderate!), and a large soup-bowl size of salad **without** dressing. For diabetics, carry almonds and munch on them with the meal. Nuts can reduce the sugar spikes created by white rice.

Very important Please carry small glass bottles of olive oil and pour it on the salad and vegetables. You will not get extra virgin olive oil in most hotels, even if it is a great hotel, because first pressed or cold pressed/extracted extra virgin olive oil is expensive. However, you can easily purchase it and carry it in check-in luggage or find a supermarket at your destination and purchase it there. Even if you don't get salad anywhere, you will be getting vegetables; have more vegetables and put three to four tablespoons of extra virgin olive oil on the vegetables to give you the anti-inflammatory, hormone-pacifying benefits.

I carry my olive oil across the world, whether I am travelling through Europe, the US, South Asia, or Australia. The only place I found pure extra virgin olive oil being served was in the cafés in Paris. Almost everywhere else, even the best hotels had second pressed oil and I can make out the difference, so I was quite disappointed. After that, I made it a rule to carry my small glass bottles or land in the city and go to the supermarket and purchase them and keep them in my hotel room or apartment (more convenient).

Mid-morning and early evening snacks Green tea with mixed nuts; all nuts are fine except cashew nuts. Rice crackers are also fine.

Green tea through the day Carry sachets with you, request hot water, and DO NOT MISS. Hot water is available on all flights; you can refill at least twice more with the same tea bag.

Emergency snacks Create two pouches containing ten almonds and ten pistachios for each day you're travelling. During the morning or early evening, if you do not find any snacks, you can munch on these along with green tea. If you manage to find snacks, these pouches can always come back. But do not forget to carry them because you need to be prepared to be nourished during emergency situations. I even carry them on the plane! Also, the moment you reach your destination, purchase apples, and add them to your emergency snacks. One apple and one pouch consisting of ten almonds and ten pistachios is a good snack to have which will keep you nourished. Along with that, you will already have your green tea sachets, and hot water is available everywhere. You can have your green tea with your nuts and your apple, and you are nourished!

Alcohol Enjoying a glass of wine with your food on holiday is fine! Unless you have serious health issues or are undergoing cancer treatment, red wine has been clinically proven to be gut-friendly, anti-inflammatory, filled with good bacteria (due to fermentation), and anti-cancer (due to resveratrol) when had in the prescribed quantities for healthy people. Everything else is fattening, bloating, and unhealthy, including hard liquor, beer, fresh juices, and even water with food. So, go ahead and enjoy! Just don't go overboard with quantities, whether it is food or alcohol.

Water Two and a half litres of water—don't forget to stay hydrated!

Sleep Eight hours of sleep—helps keep the holiday weight off!

Exercise Forty-five-minute walks during travel—roads are everywhere, so no excuses!

What to order when eating out

In a Chinese restaurant Stir-fried tofu, stir-fry vegetables, stir-fry/steamed fish. More vegetables!

In an Italian/Continental restaurant A portion of mixed leafy greens without dressing, extra virgin olive oil on the side (I always carry my small glass bottle just to be safe), a portion of grilled vegetables, grilled fish.

In an Indian restaurant The most challenging cuisine, when we are eating out, is Indian. However, even there, tandoori vegetarian kebabs like cauliflower, broccoli, mixed vegetables, and tandoori fish are available. Order whole Veg Kebabs which has vegetables rather than a Veg Hara Bhara or Veg Seekh. I would recommend eating out in north Indian restaurants less often because a lot of the food cannot be made without heavy cream, butter, and artificial colouring (remember the red Amritsari Fish Tikka?). So, try and look for other cuisines.

Everything that was harming you, if it comes back with the same intensity and frequency, will begin to harm you again.

For example, if you had a sedentary lifestyle and now with your moderate-exercise schedule, you have achieved the delicate balance in combination with the food (yes, food does not work in isolation, nor does exercise), not exercising for a month at a stretch is going to bring back many of your issues. If you skip exercise two days in a row, you should not be bending yourself out of shape in guilt. The number of days that you can go without exercise without harming yourself is three days. But then again, doing a few stretches twice a day takes just ten minutes of your time in the morning and evening. I have already shared the schedule for this; just follow it. So why skip at all?

Where food is concerned, if your dependency on excessive carbohydrates was high and you go back to eating higher quantities of carbohydrates, even if they are healthy ones, you will still end up being unhealthy. So, remember, the unhealthy habits that made you unhealthy need to be left in the past. However, indulging in these unhealthy habits occasionally is not going to harm the wonderful effort that you have put into yourself in becoming healthy in the first place. It's like a bad relationship—the more you revisit it, the more you will get sucked back into it. Having a healthy relationship means staying balanced. Staying balanced will automatically cut down cravings.

Why an elimination diet and exercise plan are the best for good health

Think of all the relationships that you have in the world. Do you end up spending time with each one of them? Why not? Because you *prioritize*. You prioritize based on those you love and those you need the most. Those you love could be your family and close circle of friends; those you need could be your colleagues and working folks. Then there is the larger circle of people who you meet probably twice a year. It is the same with your body. Your body functions on fuel and this fuel is made up of a combination of nutrients (loved ones) and calories (work folks) along with inputs from specific physical activities that help absorb these nutrients and calories. If you need only a certain amount of food, it needs to be optimal in nutrition. Enough to allow you to reap the benefits of remaining within body-weight range—not to mention high agility, freshness levels, and slowing down the ageing process as well.

For this reason, even when you are done with all the stages that will lead you to your path of being healthy and preventing diseases, going back to eating just about everything is going to be detrimental to what you have achieved till now.

A little bit of this and a little bit of that is always what dilutes the state of good health inside us.

Follow the 80:20 rule—eighty per cent of the time stick to the elimination programme and twenty per cent of the time you can indulge in some self-destructive habits! This means, from a frequency perspective, one day in a week which means four days in a month out of thirty days, you can skip exercise, eat some junk, eat low-nutrient foods or fruits, and have a little bit more of red wine. Don't do it four days in a row otherwise your inflammation levels will rise, and your mood swings will start again. From a mathematics perspective, technically you are allowed six days, which is twenty per cent of thirty, so why am I saying four days? This is because on all the other days, even if you are the most disciplined person in the world, following everything one hundred per cent would not be possible, maybe because of external circumstances beyond your control. Hence, two days get absorbed within this lack of discipline. Anyone who has followed whatever I have written has usually ended up being healthy for years to come, leaving their issues far, far behind.

Like Sadhana Ramachander from Hyderabad, who has been following a healthy lifestyle for ten years! She suddenly sent me a message: *Rachna! It's been ten years since I came to you, and you fixed me real good. Health-wise, they have been the best ten years of my post-teen life. No words to thank you.*

In June 2010, Sadhana had been running from pillar to post trying to find out the cause of her extreme unexplained pains and severe pigmentation on her legs. She was unable to walk properly due to the pain. Sadhana runs her own publishing business. For someone like her, not finding a solution was impacting her work, moods, and quality of life.

Within a few months of treatment with me, not only did she improve but she promised herself that after a year she would go on a trek. She kept working on herself and consistently stayed on the path of healing for one year. She was able to go for the trek and enjoyed every moment of it. Ten years later, she is still in the best of health because she has continued to follow the golden rules of the elimination programme.

And yes, her biological age is lower than her chronological age. Yours can be too. If you follow.

3

The Healing Foods

While all vegetables and fruits have wonderful nutrients that can reduce inflammation and fight diseases, there are some that are more powerful than the others which should be part of your elimination lifestyle as food, not supplements.

These are:

TURMERIC (HALDI)

Widely known for its anti-cancer properties due to curcumin, which is activated in the presence of pepper and oil. So, if you're using this spice in your cooking, remember to add a pinch of pepper to activate its anti-inflammatory and healing properties. Curcumin has also been found to be immuno-protective for the coronavirus[64] and aids in recovery of patients suffering from COVID-19 or any other serious viral infection, flu, frequent colds, and coughs. It is extremely heart protective and of course, it is anti-cancer[65], making it the preferred spice of everyone across the world with the number of cancer cases rising due to lifestyle and environmental reasons.

Resveratrol

Since most doctors, nutritionists, and dieticians stay away from prescribing alcohol because they cannot control quantities when people drink, and that can have a detrimental effect on health, there is not too much information dissemination about this wonderful anti-inflammatory, anti-cancer flavonoid. Resveratrol is one of the key enzymes that activates the SIRT1 gene. It can slow down the ageing process and reduce your risk of getting lifestyle diseases and cancer. In various studies, it has been shown to pacify hormones in women[66], reduce the risk for prostate cancer in men[67], reduce severe pain levels in autoimmune patients[68], dissolve deposits in the arteries which have been hardened due to age or disease[69], and reduce the risk of urinary tract infections (UTIs) in women. It is present in white wine in small quantities (not as much as in red wine) and it is not present in any other alcohol.

Foods that have resveratrol include grapes, peanuts, pistachios, blueberries, cranberries, dark chocolate, and cocoa.

Quercetin and luteolin

These are again flavonoids—luteolin, quercetin, chrysin, eriodictyol, hesperetin, and naringenin—which are anti-inflammatory, anti-tumour, and anti-viral[70]. They boost the immune system, have heart-protective properties, and balance insulin levels in the body. These flavonoids are present in celery, green peppers (capsicum), and chamomile tea. Foods specifically rich in quercetin include capers, apples, and onions. Chrysin is from the fruit of blue passionflower, a tropical vine.

Oranges, grapefruit, lemons, and other citrus fruits are good sources of eriodictyol, hesperetin and naringenin.

GARLIC

There are many large-population-based researches that have proven garlic can ward off viruses, bacterial infections including UTIs and carcinogens produced by meat cooked at high temperatures. It is extremely heart protective as well. It can lower high blood pressure, high cholesterol, and reduce hardening of arteries. Two medium-sized cloves, minced, raw, eaten twice a day is ideal. Do take the precautions of eating the raw garlic with food, so that you don't get nauseous or acidic. Remember, cooked garlic does not have anti-virus properties; cooking retains the heart-protective properties.

APIGENIN-RICH FOODS

Apigenin is mainly found in fruit (including apples, cherries, grapes), vegetables (including parsley, artichoke, basil, celery), nuts, and plant-derived beverages (including chamomile tea and red wine). It has been shown by researchers to inhibit growth in several cancers like breast, colon, skin, thyroid, and leukaemia. It has also been shown to inhibit pancreatic-cancer-cell proliferation. This compound is extremely potent as it takes away cancer cells' 'superpower' to escape death.

One of the biggest issues with cancer cells not dying is their ability to survive in most environments. Apigenin, found in what is classified as the Mediterranean vegetables, takes away the survival instinct of these cancer cells, thereby causing their death. This makes them a powerhouse to prevent cancer and lifestyle diseases[71].

The technique used by apigenin is similar to 'fishing' for the human proteins in cells that interact with small molecules available in the diet. The proteins and apigenin bind with each other. The beneficial effects of this are not limited to just cancer, as research previously proved that apigenin has anti-inflammatory properties. Therefore, by reducing inflammation, it reduces the survival capability of cancer cells.

So your plate of salad now just got bigger. Add lettuce, parsley, basil, and celery!

SEAWEED

The biggest impact is on female hormones. It can reduce hypothyroidism[72] by making the thyroid gland healthier and reduce the risk of endometriosis. It is also amazing in reducing the side effects for patients undergoing radiation. The only vegetable to have a fishy smell, seaweed's biggest anti-cancer property is to reduce the risk of hormonal cancers in women[73]. A natural component of the Japanese diet, seaweed protects us from different kinds of cancers like skin cancer and various kinds of stomach cancers[74]. Kelp and palythine, the active ingredients in seaweed, are powerful antioxidants that offer skin protection against oxidative stress, linked to cellular damage and photoaging. A diet containing kelp in seaweed lowers levels of the potent sex hormone oestradiol and can decrease the risk of oestrogen-dependent cancers like breast cancer. Prior studies have shown that Japanese women have longer menstrual cycles and lower serum oestradiol levels than their Western counterparts, which researchers say may contribute to their lower rates of breast, endometrial, and ovarian cancers. Scientists have been searching Asian diets for clues to the lower rates of cancer, with the lion's share of attention being given to soy. However, women with endometriosis and a lot of menstrual irregularities experienced significant improvement in their symptoms after three months of taking 700 mcg of seaweed capsules per day. Kelp also reduced pain associated with endometriosis and significantly lengthened the total number of days of menstrual cycles. In one of these women with high oestrogen levels, a drop in blood oestradiol levels from 600 picograms per millilitre down to 90 picograms per millilitre was seen after she included kelp in her diet.

Endometriosis, polyps, fibroids, and hormonal cancers are all a result of oestrogen overload. For women, these become the biggest hindrances towards the quality of life they can enjoy because oestrogen overload causes pain and disturbing mood swings. Bloating and unexplained weight gains are frustrating points for us to deal with, without any fault of ours. Consuming seaweed reduces all these symptoms, thereby reducing the risk of hormonal cancers. It also gives us a better quality of life because our energy levels increase, and our bloating and weight reduces. Of course, the challenge is to procure seaweed. You could get seaweed sheets from supermarkets or online and make vegetarian sushi with them (see p. 217 for recipe).

But since seaweed isn't readily available for everyone, kelp supplementation has been shown to be equally effective in reduction of oestrogen overload. Do get it prescribed by a qualified nutritional expert to reduce your risk of hormonal cancers.

GREEN TEA

The preparation and drinking of green tea are a meditative ritual, going back centuries in Japan. And that is why it is called a tea 'ceremony'. Green tea leaves are extremely potent anti-cancer and when consumed regularly, have been shown to reduce side effects of smoking, induce moderate weight loss, reduce inflammation levels, promote brain health and also protect the brain against neurodegenerative diseases like Alzheimer's and Parkinson's. When green tea extract is combined with exercise, it has shown to reduce fatty liver more effectively. It promotes gut health leading to immune-boosting benefits, is heart-protective and has been known to clinically prevent heart attacks.

With so many benefits, having three cups a day is essential for good health and prevention of lifestyle and age-related health issues. To get the right benefits, always look for leaves rather than a pouch or a sachet as the leaves have more antioxidant power. Put a bunch of leaves in a cup, pour boiling hot water over it and cover for five minutes. After five minutes, strain and drink that water. You can add organic raw honey to enhance the gut benefits. Just make sure that you do not combine your green tea with any meal; you can sip it through the day between meals.

UNSATURATED COLD FATS

Most people are deficient in these. You may be eating all your vegetables, fruits, having your green tea, and exercising well. However, the presence of cold, unsaturated fats in your meals will enhance brainpower, reduce mental agitation, and promote heart health. These are virgin flaxseed oil, extra virgin olive oil, fish oil, and the fat in nuts and seeds when eaten raw.

Make it a habit to have all the listed special foods with their therapeutic properties to ensure that you get your blast of antioxidants and flavonoids that reduce inflammation and risk for lifestyle diseases, including cancer.

4

Recipes

These recipes will help trigger your creativity in cooking scrumptious meals with healthy ingredients that can give you optimum nutrition.

SALTED PANCAKE/CHEELA/UTTAPAM-I

Makes one pancake

Ingredients

1 tbsp each of quinoa and brown rice flours
½ onion, chopped
½ capsicum, chopped
Fresh coriander, as per taste
Green chillies chopped, as per taste (optional)

Method

1. Mix all ingredients and make into batter consistency by adding water. It should pour easily but not be runny.

2. Cook like a vegetable omelette/pancake.

Note Use a 50:50 ratio of quinoa and brown rice to increase portion size.

You can make oats, brown rice and quinoa flour at home by grinding them dry and storing them in a glass container. You can store the flour separately.

Roti dough

Makes one roti

Ingredients

1 tbsp quinoa and brown rice flours (50:50 ratio)
1 tbsp of psyllium husk (Isabgol)
A pinch of ajwain (caraway seeds)
A pinch of hing (asofetida)
Sea salt or Himalayan salt, as per taste

Method

1. Mix the flours and psyllium husk together.
2. Add ajwain, hing and salt into the mixture.

Note For more options, add green chillies, a pinch of red chilli powder, fresh coriander, parsley or fresh fenugreek leaves, and chopped onions, as per taste.

Oats upma

Serves 1

Ingredients

For the oats

    3 tbsp powdered oats flour
    1 tbsp sunflower oil
    5-6 curry leaves
    1 tsp mustard seeds
    ½ onion, chopped
    ½ cup chopped vegetables (french beans, carrots, capsicum)
    Green chillies, chopped, as per taste
    A pinch of turmeric
    Whole spices (clove, cardomom, black pepper), as per taste
    2½ cup water
    Salt, as per taste

Method

1. In a bowl, take room temperature water and dissolve the powdered oats flour in it. Set aside.
2. Put a ceramic or iron pan over a medium flame. Add the oil. Once the oil is hot, add the curry leaves and let them become crisp. Add the mustard seeds and allow them to simmer for a minute.
3. Add the chopped vegetables, turmeric, salt and whole spices into the pan.
4. Stir-fry the vegetables for five minutes till they are soft but crunchy.
5. Add dissolved oats flour mixture slowly into the pan with vegetables. Add some water and boil on a high flame for five minutes.

6. Add two cups of water slowly and simmer for 7–10 minutes. Keep stirring.
7. Switch off the gas once the mixture has thickened. Serve hot.

Note All carbohydrates/protein serving sizes combined should be fifty per cent of vegetables in any form of your entire meal.

SALTED PANCAKE/CHEELA/UTTAPAM-II

Makes one pancake

Ingredients

For the rice

1 tbsp rice flour
2 tbsp oats flour
1 tbsp rice bran oil
½ onion, chopped
¼ capsicum, chopped
½ ripe tomato, chopped
2 button mushrooms, finely chopped
1 green chilli, finely chopped (optional)
2 large cloves of garlic, minced
Fresh coriander leaves, washed and chopped finely
Salt and black pepper, as per taste

For the salsa

½ onion, chopped
½ tomato, chopped

Method

1. Put the rice flour and oats flour in a bowl and add some water. Keep aside and allow it to ferment for 30 minutes.
2. Check the batter after 30 minutes. If the consistency is too thick, add some more water.
3. Put a granite saucepan on a medium flame and add the rice bran oil.
4. Put all the vegetables, green chilli, garlic, coriander, salt and pepper in the pan. Stir-fry for 2–3 minutes.
5. Reduce the flame and add the rice and oats flour mix into the vegetables. Mix and let the batter spread. The thinner it is, the more evenly you can spread it.
6. Lift the edges slightly to check that the base is golden brown, and then flip it. Make both sides crispy and golden brown.
7. To make the home-made salsa, lightly stir-fry the onions and tomatoes and mix together. Serve both together.

Note Eat only one pancake, do not exceed quantities. If eating oats results in bloating, you can replace it with brown rice, hence making a white rice and brown rice batter.

Rice Crackers

Makes 12–15 pieces

Ingredients

    1 cup brown rice
    1 cup white rice

Sea salt, as per taste

Dried herbs such as oregano, thyme, rosemary, coriander or parsley, as per taste

4 tbsp extra virgin olive oil

Method

1. Mix together the brown rice with the white rice and put in a rice cooker or pan with 6 cups of water.

2. Let the mixture overcook till it is pasty and smooth. Allow it to cool down for 45 minutes.

3. Add and mix in the sea salt and dried herbs.

4. Transfer the mixture into a mixer. Add the olive oil and water so as to get a thick consistency and blend it.

5. Take some parchment or butter paper and layer it with extra virgin olive oil.

6. Take the blended rice mixture out and spread it on the parchment or butter paper.

7. Take a knife and cut it into 2x2-inch squares—it will look like checks on butter paper.

8. Set aside and allow to dry, covered, for a couple of hours.

9. Preheat the oven to 200°C for 15 minutes. Then turn the heat down to 150°C and overturn the rice cracker squares onto an oven tray.

10. Bake for 10 minutes. Switch off the oven.

11. Let the crackers cool down completely—this should take about 45 minutes.

12. Once cooled down to room temperature, remove from the oven. The squares should now separate to give you 2-inch rice crackers.

Quinoa Cake

Serves 6

Ingredients

1 cup quinoa
2–3 apples, peeled and diced
2 pinches of clove powder
A pinch of cinnamon powder
Extra virgin olive oil for greasing
Sesame seeds for garnish
3 cups + 30 ml water

Method

1. Take quinoa and 3 cups of water and overcook it till it is pasty and smooth. Allow it to cool for 45 minutes.
2. Take the apples, and put them in a pan with the 30 ml water, clove powder, and cinnamon powder.
3. Let the mixture simmer for 1 minute and then reduce the flame. Cover the pan with a lid and leave it for 7–8 minutes till the apples are soft. Allow this to cool for 30 minutes.
4. When the quinoa and apples are both at room temperature, blend together.
5. Line an oven tray with extra virgin olive oil.
6. Heat the oven to 200°C for 10 minutes.
7. Spread the blended batter on an oven tray. Cut into 2x2-inch squares and sprinkle sesame seeds.
8. Put the tray into the oven and bake for 10 minutes. If you want it crispier, you can increase the time.
9. Allow the quinoa cake to cool in the oven for 40 minutes. After that take the tray out.

10. Serve the quinoa apple cake as a snack with green tea in the evening.

Note If you prefer more cinnamon flavour in your cakes, put in two pinches while you're preparing the batter.

MURMURA (PUFFED RICE) CHAAT WITH NUTS

Serves 1

Ingredients

3 tbsp murmura
10 crushed almonds
½ medium-sized onion, chopped
¼ medium-sized tomato, chopped
Fresh coriander, chopped
Chaat masala (or other natural flavours as per your taste)
Green chillies, chopped (optional)
A dash of lime
Salt, as per taste

Method

Toss all the ingredients together in a bowl to make bhel.

FRUIT SMOOTHIE

Serves 1

Ingredients

1 portion fruit*
50 ml almond milk (unflavoured, unsweetened Tetra Pak is fine)
2 tbsp roasted oat bran
½ tbsp cinnamon

1 tbsp powdered flaxseeds

1 spoon raw honey, optional

Method

1. Add fruit, almond milk, roasted oat bran, cinnamon, powdered flaxseeds.
2. Mix as smoothie in a mixie, add ice/cold water as per taste, add raw honey, if required.

Note If you get bloating and acidity with this, replace the roasted oats with roasted brown rice flour, the rest remains the same.

*Choose a different fruit each day. Try half an apple/5-6 medium-sized pieces of papaya/4 black grapes/4 red grapes/ 1 tbsp pomegranate/1 slice pineapple/4 berries (any kind).

Moong Sprouts

20 g moong sprouted serves 1

Ingredients

Moong beans (green grams)

Method

1. Wash whole moong beans thoroughly; first with tap water and then with hot water—do not soak the beans in hot water. This is to kill any bad bacteria or germs.
2. Soak washed moong beans in water overnight or for 12 hours—the water should be twice the amount of beans. By morning, the moong beans will double in size.
3. It will take about 24–36 hours for tiny sprouts to appear.

4. Once the sprouts have reached a desired length, cover them with water and agitate them. Drain the excess water and keep the moong beans aside.

Vegetable Sushi

Serves 6–8

Ingredients

For the rice

> 3 cups short-grain kolam rice, rinsed
> ⅓ cup rice vinegar
> Salt, as per taste

For the rolls

> 10 nori sheets, halved (available online)
> Sesame seeds, for sprinkling
> 1 cucumber
> 1 avocado
> 1 small onion
> 20 asparagus sticks, trimmed and sautéed soft
> Wasabi powder or paste, for spreading and serving on the side
> 1 romaine lettuce leaf
> Pickled ginger, for serving

Method

1. Boil the rice in a pressure cooker or a rice cooker; this gives the rice a sticky consistency.
2. In a saucepan, mix rice vinegar and one tablespoon salt and cook over medium heat.
3. Transfer the boiled rice to a large wooden bowl.

4. Drizzle a quarter of the vinegar mixture over a wooden spoon or spatula and onto the rice.

5. Fold the rice gently with the spoon to cool it and break up any clumps; be careful not to smash the grains.

6. Fold in the remaining vinegar mixture and let the rice sit for five minutes. Spread the rice evenly.

7. Cover a bamboo sushi mat with banana leaf wrap.

8. Cut a nori sheet into half and put it on the mat rough-side up.

9. Moisten your hands and scoop a handful of rice, and form it into a ball slightly larger than a lemon. Place the ball onto the nori.

10. Press the rice to spread it evenly up to the edges of the nori, moistening your fingers as you go. Sprinkle with sesame seeds.

11. Prepare the vegetables. Peel the cucumber, avocado, and onion, and slice all of them thinly. Peel the tough ends of the asparagus.

12. Carefully flip over the nori so it is rice-side down on the mat with the short-end facing up.

13. Spread a bit of wasabi paste in a line about one-third of the way up the nori—wasabi is spicy, so use it sparingly.

14. Arrange a few pieces each of lettuce, cucumber, avocado, and onion in a tight pile in the lower third of the sheet. It is fine if the vegetables spill over the edges of the nori.

15. Roll the sushi away from you with your hands, tucking in the vegetables as you go.

16. Remove the mat from under the roll and place it on top.

17. Press the roll into a compact, rectangular log using the mat to help you.

18. Slice the roll. Cut the sushi roll into 4–6 pieces.

19. Repeat with the remaining nori, rice and vegetables.
20. Serve the sushi with pickled ginger (a great fermented accompaniment) and more wasabi.

KALE AND QUINOA SALAD WITH AVOCADO

Serves 1

Ingredients

1 small sweet potato, peeled and cut into ½-inch pieces (appx. 1½ cup)
2½ tsp olive oil
½ avocado
1 tbsp lime juice
1 clove of garlic, peeled
½ tsp ground cumin
A pinch of salt
A pinch of ground pepper
1–2 tbsp water
1 cup cooked quinoa
¾ cup black beans, boiled and rinsed
1½ cups chopped kale
10–15 pumpkin seeds
1 spring onion, chopped

Method

1. Preheat oven to 200 ºC.
2. Toss the sweet potato and 1 tsp oil on a large-rimmed baking sheet.
3. Roast in the oven, stirring once halfway through, until tender, for about 25 minutes.

4. For the dressing, combine the remaining oil, avocado, lime juice, garlic, cumin, salt, pepper, and 1 tbsp water in a blender or food processor and blitz until smooth. Add another tbsp of water, if needed, to reach the desired consistency.

5. In a medium-sized bowl, combine the sweet potato, quinoa, black beans, and kale. Drizzle with the avocado dressing and gently toss the ingredients to coat evenly. Top with pumpkin seeds and spring onions.

CARROT, BEANS AND AMARANTH SABZI

Serves 3

Ingredients

½ tsp rice bran oil
1 tsp cumin
½ tsp mustard seeds
1 onion, sliced
250 g carrots
200 g beans
½ tsp turmeric powder
Salt, as per taste
1 bunch fresh amaranth leaves

Method

1. In a pan, add the oil and then add the cumin and mustard seeds. Once they start to splutter, add the onions.

2. Fry the onions till they are translucent, add the carrots, beans, turmeric, and salt, and cook for five minutes.

3. Then add the fresh amaranth leaves.

4. Add 2 tablespoons of water and cover. Leave it to simmer till it's all cooked.

5. Serve hot with 2–3 tablespoon brown rice.

PUMPKIN SOUP

Serves 4

Ingredients

1 tsp olive oil
4–5 pods garlic, sliced
1 onion, sliced
250 g pumpkin
¼ tsp cumin powder
¼ tsp coriander powder
½ tsp turmeric powder
¼ tsp cayenne pepper
Salt, as per taste
Black peppercorns, crushed for garnish
Fresh coriander leaves, for garnish
3 cups water

Method

1. In a cooker, put olive oil and then the garlic. Fry till the garlic changes colour, put the onions and sauté for some time.

2. Add the pumpkin, followed by the cumin, coriander, turmeric powder, and cayenne pepper. Sauté for some time.

3. Then add three cups of water and salt to taste. Close the lid of the cooker and allow it to cook for about 3–4 whistles.

4. Cool, then blend the mixture with a hand blender.
5. Serve the soup hot. Garnish with freshly crushed black peppercorns and fresh coriander leaves.

COFFEE WITH FENUGREEK SEEDS AND PALM JAGGERY

Serves 1

Ingredients

1 tbsp dry roasted fenugreek (methi) seeds
1 tsp palm jaggery
120 ml water
1 tsp instant coffee powder

Method

1. Add fenugreek seeds to water and boil for five minutes on a medium flame. Add palm jaggery and coffee powder to it.
2. Switch off the gas and strain the liquid. Your coffee is ready!

OMELETTE PIZZA

Serves 3–4

Ingredients

1 tbsp rice bran or any other cold-pressed oil
4 eggs
¼ cabbage
½ potato
½ carrot

1 cup spinach
Salt, as per taste
A handful of mint or coriander

Method

1. Heat the oil in a frying pan (not flat, around 2 cm depth).
2. After the oil is warm, beat 2 eggs with salt and spread evenly in the pan.
3. Chop the potatoes, cabbage, carrot, and coriander and add to the egg in an even layer. Let it cook for 1 minute.
4. Beat the remaining eggs and pour in pan, evenly covering the layer of vegetables.
5. Cook on a low to medium flame for 5 minutes. Flip the omelette once, and then again after 5 minutes.
6. Take it out of the pan after it is cooked and serve it.

DAIRY-FREE FRUIT ICE CREAM

Serves 2

Ingredients

2 portions of fruit*
500 ml almond milk, or 5 tbsp almond cream
1 handful of nuts (pistachios, almonds, etc.)
2 tsp jaggery, as a sweetener
A handful of crushed almonds

Method

1. Take any two fruits of your choice. Chop them up and refrigerate for four hours.

2. Take almond milk and beat it well using a whisk to create a cream-like consistency.
3. Now, add the chopped fruits, almond milk (or cream), and jaggery into a blender. Blend to a fine paste and refrigerate until frozen.
4. Serve the ice cream with nuts.

*1 apple/1 pineapple/1½ mango/1 cup black grapes/½ muskmelon.

Tofu Salad

Serves 1

Ingredients

2 green beans
½ capsicum
1 carrot
½ beetroot
50 g tofu
Pepper powder to sprinkle
Rock salt to sprinkle
1 tbsp flaxseed, pumpkin seed, sesame seed powder, mixed together

Method

1. Chop the vegetables into medium-sized pieces and steam them.
2. Put all the steamed vegetables in a bowl and add the tofu.

3. Adjust the seasoning according to your taste—a sprinkle of pepper powder, rock salt, and the mixed seed powder.
4. Mix well and serve.

RICE CUTLETS

Serves 2

Ingredients

1 cup cooked rice
½ cup mashed potato
1 medium onion, finely chopped
1 green chilli, chopped
2 tbsp coriander leaves
¼ tsp red chilli flakes
Salt, as per taste
3 tbsp oil

Method

1. Put all the ingredients in a mixing bowl, except the oil. Mix well. Check the taste and add more spice powders or salt if required.
2. Shape the mixture into small to medium-sized cutlets.
3. Heat the oil in a frying pan. When the oil is medium hot, place the rice cutlets in the pan.
4. When the base is lightly browned, flip them and fry the other side.
5. Once the cutlets are crisp and golden, remove from the pan and place them on a kitchen paper towel and serve.

Mackerel biryani

Serves 2-3

Ingredients

For the fish

½ kg mackerel (bangda), sliced
½ tsp salt
1 tsp red chilli powder
½ tsp turmeric powder
½ tsp coriander powder
1 tbsp garlic paste

For the masala

4 tbsp rice bran oil
3 onions, sliced
Garlic paste to taste
½ tsp red chilli powder
1 tsp coriander powder
½ tsp green chilli paste
½ tsp turmeric powder
1½ tsp salt
4–5 curry leaves
2 tbsp fresh coriander
Fresh mint leaves

For the rice

2 cups rice, soaked in water for 1 hour
6 cloves

½ tsp black cumin seeds
6 black peppercorns
One-inch piece cinnamon
2 black cardamom pods
4 tsp salt

Method

1. In a bowl mix together salt, red chilli powder, turmeric powder, and garlic paste.
2. Mix the fish with the paste and marinate for one hour. Set aside.
3. Heat oil in a pan. Add the onions and fry till medium brown.
4. Add garlic paste, red chilli powder, coriander powder, green chilli paste, and salt to the pan. Add a little water and cook for 4–5 minutes.
5. In another pan, boil the soaked rice with cloves, black cumin seeds, whole black pepper, cinnamon, black cardamom, and salt, until eighty per cent done.
6. Strain the rice.
7. In the prepared masala, sprinkle the fresh coriander leaves, curry leaves, and fresh mint.
8. Layer the rice on top of the masala. Cover the pan and simmer on a low flame for 10–15 minutes.
9. Shallow fry the marinated fish in a separate pan.
10. Remove the fish from the pan and place the fried fish on top of the rice layer.
11. Simmer for a further 5 minutes and serve hot.

Quinoa methi tikki

Serves 2

Ingredients

1 cup quinoa
1 big onion, chopped
1 or 2 green chillies, chopped
1 tbsp ginger-garlic paste
1 cup grated carrot (optional)
½ cup fenugreek (methi) leaves, chopped
1 tsp chilli powder
½ tsp cumin powder
¼ tsp garam masala (homemade)
Salt, as per taste

Method

1. Boil 3 cups water in a vessel, now add the quinoa and a little salt.
2. Boil for 15–20 minutes, and keep aside.
3. Heat a pan. Add the onions, green chillies and ginger-garlic paste. Fry until the onions turn translucent.
4. Now add the carrots and fry for 3–4 minutes.
5. Add the fenugreek leaves and fry until all the water evaporates.
6. Now add chilli powder, cumin powder, garam masala, and salt.
7. Add the boiled quinoa to this mixture. After two minutes, switch off the stove.
8. After the mixture cools, shape into small patties.

9. In a pan, heat a little oil and the shallow-fry the patties.
10. Serve the delicious quinoa methi tikki with mint chutney.

SAVOURY ITALIAN-STYLE MUFFINS

Serves 4

Ingredients

2 tbsp flaxseed
2 tbsp of water
50 g rice flour
50 g lentil or chickpea flour
1 level tsp baking soda
1 tsp gluten-free baking powder
1 cup soy/oats/almond milk yoghurt
3 tbsp rice bran oil
½ cup dried tomatoes
10-12 green and black olives
1 tbsp cider vinegar
A pinch of pepper
A pinch of salt
1 tsp each of oregano, thyme, rosemary, sage

Method

1. Preheat the oven to 180°C.
2. Mix the flaxseed and water.
3. Add flours, baking soda, baking powder, yoghurt and oil successively. Mix well with a whisk.

4. Separate the dough, and put black olives and tomatoes in half of the dough and sprinkle the herbs in the other half so you have 2 different types of muffins.

5. Bake for about 15 minutes—the baking time depends on the size of your muffin pans so watch out!

APPLE AND FIG COBBLER

Serves 4

Ingredients

4 large apples of Golden or Himachal variety, peeled, cored and cut into coarse cubes
6 fresh figs, chopped
100 g rice flour
50 g chickpea flour
40 g almond powder
100 g plant-based butter, or margarine
80 g brown sugar

Method

1. Preheat your oven to 180° C.
2. Cook the apple cubes and figs in a saucepan over low heat for about 10 minutes until the fruit softens.
3. Transfer the fruit to an ovenproof dish or individual ramekins.
4. Pour the flour, margarine, sugar and coconut into a mixing bowl.
5. Mix until it forms a lumpy dough.
6. Cover the fruit with the dough and bake in the oven for 25 minutes. Serve warm.

Rainbow Buddha bowl (vegan and gluten-free)

Ingredients

3-4 broccoli florets
1 tbsp cornniblets
3-4 cauliflower florets
Turmeric powder to taste
5-6 mushrooms, sliced
Olive oil
A handful of spinach leaves
½ cup boiled foxtail millets
¼ cup boiled chickpeas
1 tbsp mixed seeds
1 tsp mixed berries
1 tbsp fermented beetroot
1 tbsp purple cabbage sauerkraut
1 spring onion, chopped
¼ cucumber, sliced
½ tomato, sliced
Salt, as per taste

For the dressing/sauce

7–8 dates, soaked
1-inch piece tamarind, soaked
Salt, as per taste
¼ tsp roasted cumin powder
Water for soaking/blending

Method

1. Lightly steam the broccoli and corn. Keep aside.
2. Steam the cauliflower in water infused with half teaspoon turmeric powder. Keep aside.
3. In a pan, sauté the mushrooms in olive oil. Add salt. Keep aside.
4. Similarly, sauté the spinach, foxtail millets and set aside.
5. Now, sauté the chickpeas, add some salt and turmeric powder.
6. Once everything is ready, arrange everything on a platter side by side.
7. Sprinkle the seeds, berries, and spring onion.
8. To make the date and tamarind sauce, soak the deseeded dates and tamarind separately. Take out the pulp.
9. Blend the soaked dates and tamarind in a blender with salt, jeera and some water to make a smooth sauce.
10. Serve the vegetables with the date and tamarind sauce.

SUPER SEEDS FRUIT AND NUT SMOOTHIE (VEGAN AND GLUTEN-FREE)

Serves 1

Ingredients

10 gm each of pumpkin, sunflower, watermelon, muskmelon, flaxseed and chia seeds, powdered
10 almonds
2 walnuts
5 cashews
10 raisins, or as per taste
2 dates

1 portion fruit*
50 ml water (increase water if you want thinner consistency)

Method

Blend together all the ingredients in a high-speed blender and serve cold.

*3 strawberries/1 apple/5-7 blueberries

ZOODLES WITH A CASHEW MORINGA PESTO (VEGAN AND GLUTEN-FREE)

Ingredients

1 large zucchini, spiralized
Handful of cherry tomatoes
6 cape gooseberries, halved (optional)
1 carrot, spiralized
1 cucumber, spiralized
1 tomato, chopped lengthwise
Pecans and walnuts, crushed
A bunch of microgreens

For the pesto

¼ cup raw cashews
½ tsp moringa leaf powder
2 cloves of garlic
Olive oil
1 tbsp lemon juice
Rock salt, as per taste
Black pepper, as per taste

Method

1. Mix all pesto ingredients and blend in a blender.

2. Lightly cook the pesto and zucchini in a pan.
3. Add the tomatoes and cape gooseberries.
4. Garnish with carrots and cucumber. Top with the nuts and microgreens to serve.

GRILLED CORIANDER FISH

Ingredients

Any oily fish, cut into 5-6 medium-sized pieces
A handful of coriander leaves
10–12 cloves of garlic
2 tbsp rice bran oil
½ tsp powdered black peppercorns
Juice of half lemon (optional)
Sea salt to taste

Method

1. In a mixer, add coriander leaves, garlic cloves, oil, and crush to a coarse mixture. You can also make a paste by adding a little water.
2. In a bowl, add the fish pieces, coriander mixture and sprinkle the black pepper and salt.
3. Brush a grill pan with a little oil and put in the fish pieces. Grill both sides for 5–7 minutes each.
4. If using a microwave oven, preheat the oven setting to 190º C and grill for 10 minutes on each side.
5. Pour extra virgin olive oil over the grilled fish and serve with coriander or mint chutney.

Additional recipes contributed by Neha Bali, Fatima Mirza, Akhil Neerugatti, Farah Choudhry, Manasa Kiran, Camille Tomat, Shefali Batra, Rajshree Deo.

Part 5

The
New Order

*Drive yourself
to a higher consciousness.*

1

Last Human Standing

Chhachhi Sir or Mr H.B.S. Chhachhi, is 91 years old. He has been an educator all his life, teaching kids for forty-plus years before retiring. He was the principal of Hindalco Vidya Niketan (now rechristened Aditya Birla Public School), Renukoot, and is not only still remembered by his students but also revered.

If I had to look for a living example on everything being amalgamated for a wonderful quality of life and longevity, it is this man. He unknowingly has lived it. I have observed him live his life the way he does for the last twenty-seven years, so he is my favourite study subject on longevity. He does not have any lifestyle disease, has not been operated upon for anything serious, and his mind is razor-sharp. The telltale signs of ageing at 91 years are his frailty, a hunch and loss of hearing. You can see him most days sitting at his desk, reading something, and making notes. He has innumerable notebooks filled with notes because whatever interesting stuff he finds in the books he reads, he jots it down. He is my father-in-law. Daddy.

At mealtimes, he is a frugal eater and has always been. I have been through conversations with everyone in the family on how he will not, *repeat not*, take a second helping. He has a reasonable breakfast with eggs, a small lunch with fruits and yoghurt, a munchy evening tea with half a sandwich and a frugal dinner with a few spoons of vegetables, one rolled up roti and a few spoons of some curry. This curry could be the curry of a dish made or a light-yellow lentil, but just a few spoons. He sleeps in the afternoon and sleeps on time at night to wake up fresh at 5 a.m. every day. He fights with the household help to wash the utensils because he loves doing it himself. Always has. He's a bit of a cleanliness freak and cannot stand injustice. If he feels short-changed by someone, I have seen him go up to young robust men and yell at them. He is unaware of his own frailty at that time because he is strong in his mind—that's his image of himself. So, he will be fearless in his aggression if something is not right.

And his daily indulgence, *daily*, is a cup of coffee at 11.30 a.m. with 90 ml Baileys Irish Cream. Every single day. During the lockdown when his supply ran out and wine shops were closed, he was ready to fight with anybody for his 90 ml shot.

Everything that I have mentioned in the book can be related to him in terms of mental health, sharpness of the mind, the ageing process of the human body and how to keep it alive. Daddy is my biggest learning. He has been practising all his life what we have learnt through science and holistic nutrition. Let us break it down and do a little recap based on his life.

Recap

We have an anti-ageing gene that gets activated when we eat twenty per cent less than our hunger I have talked about the SIRT1 gene in my book. And each person I interviewed and my observation with Daddy is that this gene is activated. Otherwise, how many 91-year-old people do you know who have not had a lifestyle disease or a major surgery any time in their life?

I have also seen that eating frugal meals is much more beneficial than two meals a day, as is being practised by a lot of people now. It keeps blood sugar levels steady, metabolism high and nutrients intake consistent. He is famous for being stubborn about small quantities of meals and snacks in the family, extended family and even his student's circle. Nobody can influence him to eat more than what he has been eating forever. While eating twenty per cent less, Daddy has one meal and four snacks a day—by no standards will any normal person call his lunch and dinner a full meal. He only has one reasonably okay meal, which is breakfast. For anybody who has been brainwashed into skipping breakfast, this is one of the biggest causes for belly fat, hypothyroidism, fatigue, and brain fog. When you are starving yourself, your body will go into fat storage. Skipping meals is one of the biggest reasons for the slow thyroid secretion in women. In teenagers, it can cause hormonal fluctuations and weight gain along with a sluggish brain that makes it difficult to understand lessons in school.

Then he has a snack at 11.30 a.m., mainly his coffee with Irish cream along with a couple of bites of a few nuts or half a piece of chocolate. Then, a frugal lunch of fruits and yoghurt which would be a snack for most people. Then another side snack at 4.30 p.m. and an equally frugal dinner by 7.30 p.m. By habit, since he was an adult, he has been doing natural intermittent fasting by eating his last meal at 7.30 p.m. and eating only fourteen hours later at 9.30 a.m. the next day. The fad about intermittent fasting has its basis in giving your digestive system a break just like you are giving your brain and body a break during the rest and repair process. Eating an early dinner naturally creates this and you don't have to starve at breakfast and combat the negative effects of skipping breakfast.

The mind controls the ageing process His ability to copiously read, research, and jot down new learnings is creating neural pathways on a regular basis, keeping him razor-sharp. He may have lost his hearing, but his mind is intact. Everybody has tried to convince him to wear a hearing aid, but he refuses. During social gatherings, when somebody is making a speech, he will nudge me and say, 'I don't have to listen to this bakwaas (nonsense). Therefore, I don't wear a hearing aid; I don't want to hear things that irritate me.' And he says this with a twinkle in his eye and starts giggling. He keeps the toxicity out voluntarily.

The fact that, in his own mind, he is still that strong, aggressive person makes him feel youthful. It is when we adopt a defeatist attitude towards facing problems that we lose the battle. There are so many people ageing well, but they keep themselves young by learning new things, being in the company of younger people and keeping themselves abreast of whatever interests them. With Daddy too, meeting old students, nourishing his brain with new books, learning new words every day—his dictionary is his other companion—keeps the brain ticking and alive. With an alive brain, the mind will refuse to accept ageing as a pessimistic and defeatist process. You will age but in a happier mental state.

A small amount of indulgence is necessary There are many studies that have proven that moderate consumption of alcohol leads to longevity, a healthier heart, even and steady blood pressure, and better moods. In fact, moderate alcohol consumption is a natural blood thinner. Ronnie has his two small whiskies, and Ronnie is 81. His heart is good. And so is Daddy's. That large shot of Baileys Irish Cream seems to be doing the trick.

Studying 7,697 people between age 45 and 64 who were non-drinkers and who were participating in the Atherosclerosis Risk in Communities (ARIC) study[75] over a ten-year period, medical researchers found that six per cent of the subjects began moderate alcohol consumption (one drink a day or fewer for women and two drinks a day or fewer for men) during the follow-up period. After four years of follow-up, the new moderate drinkers had a thirty-eight per cent lower chance of developing cardiovascular disease than their non-drinking counterparts. Even after adjusting for physical activity, BMI, demographic, and heart-risk factors, this difference persisted. While I advocate only red wine because of its anti-inflammatory properties and activating the anti-ageing gene—hence being doubly rewarding—it seems that science supports any alcohol as long as it is in small quantities[76].

Sleep and rest, rejuvenate and repair Each one of us fall short on the sleep parameters, not realizing that the deficit of repair work will continue to pile up and make degenerative changes in our DNA if we don't fix it. Eight to nine hours of sleep is recommended by sleep doctors, but I don't know too many corporate executives or schoolgoing kids who follow this. But I do know this 91-year-old man without any diseases sleeping a full night and catching a snooze in the afternoon. His health, mind, and sense of humour are all intact.

Keep the sh*t out That is what he does by choosing not to wear the hearing aid. And even before he lost his hearing, his students remember him to be a no-nonsense guy. He would be fond of the mischievous lot but intolerant of injustice. It is important to nurture ourselves with what we do, which he does with his reading. When he began to lose his hearing, he did try to wear a hearing aid but, in those times, they used to generate a static sometimes that hurt his ear. He decided against it because his inability to hear was not affecting his quality of life. This is called the selective process; it aids in self-preservation and keeping emotional toxicity out. If Daddy doesn't like you, you will know. If he is fond of you—and he will be if you are weird or quirky because those people interest him—again, you will know. He keeps life simple and his communication simple. His mind is crystal clear. There is no space for uncertainty, doubt, or anguish. All these cause a lot of stress and emotional trauma in our lives. There are very few people who are on sure ground and it comes with knowledge and confidence. Yes, it is difficult to achieve this kind of clarity; however, if you were true to your work and have depth in your knowledge, you will always be on sure ground. Too many people we know will take shortcuts, run after greed, hide things, or not be thorough in their work, or deep in their relationships. Even if it has worked for you, your heart knows that you are short-changing yourself. Don't do it. It can cause you your peace of mind. If you keep the toxicity out, and remain deep and true, the clarity will automatically come.

Meditation has clear cognitive benefits Whenever anyone is advised to meditate, and I advise a lot of people to do it, it is for people who are stressed out. It is for people who cannot focus on one task at a time and cannot be in the present and focusing on what they are thinking, doing, or reading. All the clinical data on the wonderful and beautiful effects of meditation are on people with cancer, heart disease, depression, anxiety, chronic stress, emotional conflict, or unrest. It is to help them overcome their negative thoughts by focusing on the here and now to calm the agitation in the brain and reduce inflammation. By meditating, reduction of inflammation repairs the DNA and reduces the ageing process. But for people who can focus on a singular task and are mindful, any habit that inculcates a meditative state has the same results as practising meditation. It could be music for somebody if they are not thinking of twenty different things and can focus *only* on the music. It could be sitting by the beach and watching the waves and the sunset for another person who *only* has gratitude for the sunset and the vast ocean, no other thoughts. The activity of meditation must be performed daily for us to continue the repair process or reduce ageing of the brain and body. Daddy doesn't need meditation because his copious reading *every day* makes him focused on one activity at a time and he already has the mindfulness.

The purpose of meditation is to leave behind your stresses and only focus on one thought or one task.

Of course, Chhachhi Sir, or Daddy, is naturally like this. What if you are not? I have extensively put steps on how to achieve the balance in the previous chapter. This balance cannot be achieved by the mind till the body is not nourished in a balanced manner. That is why the steps to achieve the physical balance of nutrients, moderate exercise, and breathing techniques will finally lead us to the path of meditation. These steps will make our mind calm and reduce the fluctuations. It is only then that we can naturally focus on a single task at a time without our thoughts being dissipated.

So, the first step for those of you who are by nature different but would like to achieve the real benefits of meditation, is getting your physical nourishment in place. I know many people tell me they meditate every day, but obviously they do not understand the meaning of meditation because it does not reflect in their behaviour. A meditative mind, whether you do meditation or not, is going to be without conflict. Meditation makes us accept and love ourselves the way we are. And when we start doing that, all conflicts disappear. We choose what is best for us and our loved ones and stop taking shortcuts.

Yes of course, if you're a working professional, you will say that you cannot spare the time to first get your physical balance to be ready for meditation. But Sivakumar Surampudi (Shiv) does not agree.

As a corporate leader, he chose to get this balance.

When Shiv came to me, his body language was closed. He had some health issues, some reports were out of range, he had severe knee pain, hypertension and was forty kilos overweight.

At the age of 57, 114 kilos, his work meant twenty days of travel every month. As group head of agribusiness and IT at ITC, he is leading a large team and a lot of responsibility was on his shoulders.

It was not that he was unaware of his health issues and had not tried earlier. But lack of time and a packed schedule along with travel always affected the consistency of input. He and his colleague and buddy Nazeeb Arif, head of corporate affairs, ITC, decided to get healthier together in 2017. They would check into a health centre for a week, lose weight, go on with life as normal and gain it right back. This pattern continued for almost two years till Shiv began to get chronic knee pain and realized that his travel would be affected and hence, his work output would suffer. When Nazeeb reached out to me, he urged Shiv to do the same.

So here we were, in my clinic on a cool December afternoon in Bandra West, Mumbai. I had to step out for an emergency and Shiv had to wait, and he was not used to waiting. We sat and discussed for forty minutes what my programme would target and how it would systematically reduce inflammation and, by virtue of reducing inflammation, how his knee pain would ease, hypertension would disappear, reports would come back to normal, and his weight loss would be accelerated. Shiv nodded, seeming extremely unconvinced and said, 'What about my travel?' I reassured him that we will deal with it. And so, he signed up. That was 3 December 2019.

Six months later, during our video session, after having lost thirty-five kilos and reversing his knee pain and hypertension, Shiv confessed, 'I never thought we could reach here.' He was mentally prepared to lose ten kilos and 'see how it goes'. But today, when I told him that he needs to reach the magical number of seventy-five kilos, he laughed and said, 'Today I believe you. When we met on 3 December, in my mind I was like, that's not going to happen.'

The first fourteen days of his plan, from 4 December through 18 December, Shiv not only travelled crazily, but he was in one city for not more than a day. I would ask him which hotel he was staying at and recommend food from the menus listed. In those first fifteen days, he lost four kilos. And then there was no looking back.

Through the lockdown, when everyone lamented their lack of choices, he stuck to the limited choices available, but refused to deviate from food groups. Exercise was a challenge with crazy back-to-back Zooms, but we worked out spurts of fifteen-minute exercises spread through the day to keep his BMR high and inflammation low. Circulation was key so water was a big focus.

'I think what really worked was the consistency,' he confesses. He had never been given the tools to be consistent before. 'What you did with me was like management pillars—inspire, enable, track.' And then, Shiv broke it down:

Inspire he was inspired to join my programme because my focus was understanding what was happening inside his body via his biomarkers and symptoms and my treatment was holistic. I broke his goal down with him into smaller milestones. Even though I talked about the end goal of forty kilos, which he was disbelieving of, I told him that he needs to focus on ninety-nine kilos. I explained to him that I could not give him heavy exercising till he reached that goal weight as his heart would be at risk. And so, along with gentle and low exercise, we used nutrition to achieve ninety-nine. After that, the next goal was ninety-five, eighty-nine and then eighty-five. 'The smaller milestones seem achievable and here we are, we have achieved them.' Breaking down any goals always makes them less threatening and makes sequential following of instructions easier.

Enable 'You gave me a twenty-four-hour chart which had very little flexibility, whether it was food, sleep, water or exercise. It made sure that I got into a twenty-four-hour rhythm and enabled me to eat as per the charts when I was travelling. It was also easy for my secretary and family to understand and implement and everyone supported me in this period,' says Shiv, evidently grateful to the ecosystem around him that made it all happen. And I have seen this with other clients and patients of mine as well—when the chart is watertight, the results are miraculous. When a lot of people shift from the chart to dos and don'ts, many people slip. But since we cannot live life going from one chart to the other, I give watertight instructions of dos and don'ts as well. 'Yes, this continuation of rhythm is what made consistency happen,' shares Shiv. One of the boons of the lockdown was that he could walk in small spurts at home before each meal. And that is something I advocate to everybody. People who work out for one hour every day and are sitting for twelve hours after that are not as successful in achieving holistic health with a healthy heart, healthy joints, lower inflammation levels, and being disease-free.

Whether it is milestones for health goals or milestones broken down into smaller elements, doing everything in moderation brings inconsistency. It is always easier to say, I can spare time for fifteen minutes of walking before lunch, and much more difficult to say that I will spare one hour in the evening. So many senior corporate executives do not even have that one hour to spare. Hence, enabling them to achieve holistic well-being by breaking down exercise into smaller parts keep circulation and BMR high.

Track This is a crazy one. 'What you measure is what you can manage,' says Shiv. 'You asked me to give you daily weight updates and even though it was not your singular focus, it kept me on track. Every evening I would eat, I would be mindful of my quantities because the weight the next morning would determine the kind of emoticon you would send me!'

We both laughed at this, and he reminded me of the kind of emoticons I would keep sending him. The most dreaded was when there was no movement in weight.

With thirty-five kilos gone, no knee pain, Shiv's moods are jovial and stress management capabilities are much more efficient. He consciously takes out time to sleep more, something that the corporate world robs you of. He is a shining example of everything going against him and he still managed to not only stay on track but achieve his difficult health goals. He could have hidden behind the excuses of extensive travel, long work hours, too much sitting, no time for exercise, or breath work ... But he did not. He found a solution every time he reached a stumbling block. Like I have said earlier, asking never hurts and often, the universe listens to what you are asking for and conspires to give it to you. And this is what happened with Shiv too.

Shiv's inherent nature is extremely social enterprise driven (he did his first job with the famous Dr Kurien at Anand after graduating from IRMA). So even the work that he does today as head of the Agri businesses and the organic gardening done at home points towards sustainable living.

Chhachhi Sir/Daddy, Shiv and so many others are from a previous generation.

But there is a growing breed of young people across the world who are choosing this conscious living over materialistic dreams. Nurturing themselves and the environment around them is interlinked for them. Being healthy and expressing gratitude are both important for well-being. And the next generation truly believes that the journey of life and its experiences lived in a sustainable manner are more important than the corporate bigwig trappings.

2

The Torch Bearers of Consciousness

A consciousness for self and the Earth is rising not just amongst individuals but also organizations. Sustainable living is good for us, provides us and the earth with the holistic nutrition required to nurture and nourish, and the biggest outcome is gratitude. Sustainability for these young torchbearers means both things: sustainability of our own quality of life in sync with nature, not against it. When I look around me, I have met many of them.

Camille is 27 years old, is French but knows three languages, and was a food technology professional. But she decided to come to Mumbai, to learn yoga. When I asked her why, she simply said with mental clarity not common in people her age, 'It has been a long time since I wanted to explore yoga. I wouldn't have done it outside of India because it originates from there.' After yoga, she decided to do a holistic health coach certification programme and began her career as a healer.

Aradhna is 23 years old. She studied design communication and wanted to be a photographer. During her diploma, at the age of 19, she developed chronic back issues and every photography project she did, her back would hurt even more. After running from orthopaedics to neurologists to getting MRIs done, she was overmedicated but did not find relief. She had to give up photography and completely rest for a few months without her laptop, camera, or phone. The side effects of medications and the sedentary lifestyle due to pain triggered PCOS. Struggling with PCOS side effects, acne, weight gain and hair fall, she refused to take hormonal tablets and medications for PCOS; instead, she turned to my anti-inflammatory nutrition programme and her pain levels reduced by eighty per cent. Her PCOS reports became negative in a span of just five months. And gentle yoga, a part of my plan, helped her lose the weight she had gained. But the acne persisted, and she learnt to live with it.

Not being able to pursue her passion to be a photographer, she wasn't disheartened for too long. During her rest period, she discovered a new profession—to be a sommelier. She became a French wine scholar but refused to take up a job. She was offered sommelier jobs by exclusive wine restaurants and a prestigious five-star hotel chain in Mumbai. But she said no. 'I'm very clear about my quality of life. I like to keep normal work hours, spend time with my friends and family and these kinds of jobs mean that you have to be out till 1 a.m. It doesn't work for my priority of things.'

She started her own company and began doing wine-experience events. During the lockdown, wine experiences diminished and so she turned to Yin Yoga. 'I had been doing yoga as a kid and don't have much value for Power Yoga or any fast form of yoga,' she confesses. 'A lot of people are not aware of their own body and I chose Yin Yoga, where you hold the pose and become aware of how that part of your body and muscles are feeling. It is about awareness of our bodies and them being in sync with our mind and soul.' It was with Yin Yoga that her acne disappeared. Even though she was clinically negative for PCOS, the lingering symptoms like acne and moodiness persisted. But Yin Yoga, a passive form of yoga which activates the feminine energy, helped her completely reverse her health issues.

Today, Aradhna is teaching Yin Yoga to women with hormonal issues and is also doing sessions on yoga and wine. 'I am combining the benefits of yoga with the benefits of a glass of wine and healthy food,' she says. 'It's fun. We have to enjoy the journey. I have left my moodiness and acne behind. I'm not only loving this but also experiencing gratitude from those I help,' she says.

I have not met a single soul who experiences gratitude and has long bad moods. It is when we overcome and expel the devil of toxins in our minds and bodies that the real repair work begins in the form of feeling lucky and appreciative of who we have and what we have in our lives. These toxins could be inflammation, excess food, drink, tobacco, drugs, side effects of medications, and stress; they can all be released by the path of balanced holistic nutrition.

As individuals are realizing the importance of holistic nutrition to prevent, manage or reverse the conditions and turning away from toxic medications, there are organizations which are also being awakened. The large number of employee-sickness days, low productivity, and midlife crisis due to burnout has made just a handful of people across the globe pre-empt and want to fix this problem. Organizations are realizing that healthier employees are more efficient employees, and this impacts their bottom line positively.

And helping them is Andrew Hewitt. He helps companies adapt to 'care' values via his company, Game Changers 500 (GC500). GC500 profiles the world's top purpose-driven organizations and consults with them to work towards good deeds and sustainability-driven outcomes.

Andrew is not your run-of-the-mill entrepreneur running after valuations, his next billion, and that big car in the driveway. Having a conversation with him is calming, unhurried, and therapeutic. His daily meditation routine and yoga practice emit an energy that makes organizations realize the futility of running after profit at any cost. 'I am a yogi, and my sister is a Christian,' he confesses. 'And our values are still the same.' At 37, his emotional maturity level is much higher. And that is why he is in demand with organizations that seek to change their culture, their employee focus, the way they reward, and measure profits.

'A few years out of college and so many of my friends had already burnt out,' shares Andrew. 'These were the same guys who were hungry to join the Fortune 500 companies, the global giants, and climb the ladder of success. But what I saw in my friends was burnout and depression.' Andrew launched GC500 in 2010 at Harvard's Igniting Innovation Summit.

So, what does GC500 do? Simply put, it is an alternate system to Fortune 500 companies and ranks the world's top *mission-driven* businesses in order of their mission, purpose and impact on employee health, and sustainability. It pushes companies to care.

RACHNA CHHACHHI

The largest impact of wellness and a holistic balance can be achieved at the workplace. Everybody goes to work. Everybody needs to work. Why must they not enjoy what they do? 'After the 2008 financial debacle, a lot of young people were disillusioned and companies were not being able to hire bright minds,' says Andrew. 'They invited me to help them hire talent. But organizations should hire people who are purpose driven and not driven; the change needs to come at that level.'

Andrew's company consults with traditional and social enterprise organizations on how they can be the game changers for sustainable living. But like I have seen with my patients and you may have experienced it yourself, till the time the consultative process is on, the impact of changing for good happens. When the active consulting is gone and guidelines are given to continue the changed lifestyle or, in the company's case, the changed philosophy and culture, there are slip-ups back to traditional systems.

Like I did with Shiv and thousands of people I have treated, GC500 also has a system to inspire, enable, and track. Some organizations already had this, and others needed to adapt. 'The difficult part is to get a large and old organization to change. We managed to do it with some and with others we failed, but I see that as a learning,' shares Andrew. His project with Unilever was very successful where his company consulted on product innovations that are also sustainable. What they realized was that the good for the Earth and sustainable products this year are also more profitable, hence, Unilever's portfolio for such products is growing. However, GC500 could not achieve the same thing with Kraft. 'It was eight months of hard work with no results. Ultimately, the company was merged with Heinz and the then CEO retired for good after making US$19.5 million,' says Andrew with a sigh. 'I had to go back to the drawing board because I literally had the carpet pulled from under me on this one.'

But he has been lucky to be in touch with organizations which promote sustainable living. Fabindia, Organic India, Guayakí teas, Barry-Wehmiller, and Google are some of the companies that inspired Andrew because their purpose is aligned with caring for the world.

But the difference is, this focus is via benefit for all including the planet.

So, what prompted Andrew to start GC500? 'The year I began, one of my friends, who was working at KPMG and had a dream job at the age of 30, committed suicide. Depression killed him.' This incident, and seeing other friends struggle with the bitter reality of their big dreams, anguished Andrew. What made things worse was that after his friend was no more, another friend of his, Mike, being as disturbed as Andrew, approached his HR saying that things will have to change if employees were to be saved. And his HR manager told him, 'Nothing will change. You will quit from here and go to another organization, it is the same.' This futility of the corporate system shocked both Andrew and Mike and Mike quit his job and joined Andrew to start GC500 to create what Andrew calls an 'alternative plan'.

GC500 has been in operations for the last ten years and there have been some very good experiences and some learnings. There are some wonderful organizations which have all the parameters and are a shining example of benefit for all. The parameters are:

1. An inspiring and comfortable employee culture.
2. Products which do not harm the environment and Earth.
3. There is profit, but not at the cost of employee health or sustainability.
4. The organization *cares*. This care can result in financial wins too. As per WHO, research has demonstrated that workplace health initiatives can help reduce sick leave absenteeism by twenty-seven per cent and healthcare costs for companies by twenty-six per cent.

What makes Andrew different from other 'successful' people is his uncompromising stand on the good values and ethics. For the world around him as well as for himself as an individual. If you look at his background and his daily habits, his calmness is proof of the life that he leads. Born to achiever parents who were authors and speakers and having attended one of the top colleges in Canada, Andrew was quickly disillusioned with the education system and began a venture to help college students find their purpose. The venture did so well that at the age of 24, he had made his money. But he had not bargained for this success. 'In the eyes of people around me, I was a successful entrepreneur, but this was not my definition of success,' he says. 'I was getting into meditation and yoga and I realized that I was a product of the ecosystem and I did not believe in this ego-driven ecosystem. I needed to get out and build an alternate ecosystem.' So, at the age of 24, he bought a one-way ticket to Costa Rica and left. And it was in Costa Rica that the idea of GC500 started germinating.

Today, GC500 is driving the change for sustainable profitability. 'I am not saying don't make money, but also care for your people, for the planet.' Organizations have that responsibility. You may not attend a weekend webinar on meditation, but you go to work every day. And your organization knows that you are there, and it can help you by incorporating these values and habits at the most captive space and time—in the office hours. The result will be healthier, happier employees and higher productivity.

As we draw to a close with my discussion and this book, Andrew tells me that he loves nature and basking in the stillness of the forest. Very often, he takes out his electric mountain bike on a ride to soak in the natural environment. I asked him what his guilty pleasures are. 'I am a cookie monster!' he laughs and tells me. Other than that, he's not very fond of alcohol but tulsi tea does the job beautifully. He meditates every day and the stillness of nature brings a gratitude which keeps him grounded. It's that word again—gratitude. Which makes us complete. We cannot feel gratitude till we are not physically and emotionally in sync with ourselves.

WHAT IS THE NEW ORDER?

Whether you look at Camille, Aradhna or Andrew, all three are from different parts of the world but with one focus— *unhurried sustainable living*. This wise Generation Y realizes the impact of stress on leading a hurried life, running after materialistic dreams, and taking away from the Earth. There are millions like them, refusing to bow down to the conventional definition of success and healthcare. They have rejected an established order at two levels—for their own health and for their work. Because the current order compromised quality of life and peace of mind in some ways.

They are the torchbearers of consciousness and are leading companies, individuals, and the Earth into being in sync with body, mind, and spirit for themselves, those they consult with, and with the Earth. *They feel responsible.*

When we start to feel unwell, the responsibility for feeling well is ours and not the medical system's or the doctor's. Equipped with the correct knowledge of balanced physical and emotional nutrition, we can achieve a disease-free status which increases our quality of life drastically and makes us enjoy each day. The beautiful results of being on this path for all the people I have interviewed and treated are: higher energy, joy in the every day, and gratitude. At the end of the day, it is not just you who needs that. The world needs to increase its wellness quotient at the individual, organizational and planet level. And it is only then that we can all be healthier and happier people. And that change starts with you.

Be the change.

Gratitude

Thank you, Vikram, for editing this book with passion, commitment, and a sense of wonder. You haven't lost the senior editor instinct. Your sensitivity makes you a higher man than most men can hope for. As my partner in love, life, and friendship, your compassion and goodness make me respect you just a bit more, every day.

This book is a much better version of the original because of Sonal Nerurkar who got completely stressed out while making it shine, and then, used the breathing techniques in the book to calm herself down!

I have never met you, Ritu, but your positivity in expressing my yoga poses so beautifully was meditative. Ritu Jain is pursuing fashion media communication. At 22, she is one of the torchbearers of this generation in demonstrating a life of balance. Her minimalism is reflective of leaving behind toxicity of a world created by greed and holding. She lets go with her art. You will be lucky if she agrees to work with you. You can reach her at ritujain.hi@gmail.com to benefit from her energy.

My sincere thanks to all my partner healers who patiently waited for me to finish this book and learnt to become independent without their Mama healer constantly being around.

A big thank you to all my patients and clients who put up with my delays in email and chart responses.

And finally, for Aradhna, who is leading this new order. Thank you for changing my perspective as a person, as your mother. Your emotional sensitivity gives me hope to heal millions burdened with avarice.

About the Author

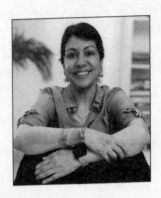

Rachna Chhachhi is PhD, Holistic Nutrition, certified Nutritional Therapist and Holistic Cancer Coach, WHO-certified in malnutrition. She has her own practice for cancer, autoimmune and lifestyle diseases across 27 countries under *RachnaRestores* and has devised an online holistic health coach certification programme which is internationally accredited. Globally, over 200+ holistic health coach practitioners have been certified by her coaching programme.

As a certified cancer coach in both holistic cancer from BeatCancer and Cancer Metastasis from Johns Hopkins University, Rachna also heads the Asia wing of BeatCancer. org (The Center for Advancement in Cancer Education), a non-profit global organization headquartered in Pennsylvania, USA. She carries forth the mission of BeatCancer across Asia.

Rachna has been a health writer for twenty years and has been a columnist with *BusinessWorld*, *Business Today*, *Outlook Business* and *Times of India* (TOI Blogs). She authored her first book *Restore* which helps people overcome lifestyle diseases by restoring their health. Her second book, *You Can Beat Cancer*, was launched on World Cancer Day in 2020. *Alive!* is Rachna's third book.

When anyone asks her about her personal *mantra* for good health, she just lovingly stares at her plants and her hot cup of green tea.

Notes

1. Our World in Data, 'Cause of deaths for 50 to 69 year olds, world, 2017', accessed 18 January 2021; https://ourworldindata. org/grapher/causes-of-death-in-50-69-year-olds

2. Clintoria R. Williams et al., 'Zinc Deficiency Induces Hypertension by Promoting Renal Sodium Reabsorption', *American Journal of Physiology–Renal Physiology*, 2019; doi: 10.1152/ajprenal.00487.2018

3. Medical News Today (blog), 'Why self-love is important and how to cultivate it', accessed 18 January 2021; https:// www.medicalnewstoday.com/articles/321309#The-ills-of-perfectionism

4. Lauren Gaydosh et al.,'The Depths of Despair Among US Adults Entering Midlife', *American Journal of Public Health*, 109 (5), 2019: 774; doi: 10.2105/AJPH.2019.305002

5. Evilena Anastasiou et al., 'Infectious disease in the ancient Aegean: Intestinal parasitic worms in the Neolithic to Roman Period inhabitants of Kea, Greece', *Journal of Archaeological Science: Reports*, 2017; doi: 10.1016/j.jasrep.2017.11.006

6. Medical News Today (blog), 'What is modern medicine?', accessed 18 January 2021; https://www.medicalnewstoday.com/ articles/323538

7. Loudon, Irvine, 'A brief history of homeopathy', *Journal of the Royal Society of Medicine*, 99 (12), 2006: 607–10; doi:10.1258/jrsm.99.12.607

8. Andrew Weil Center for Integrative Medicine (blog), 'What is Integrative medicine?', accessed 18 January 2021; https://integrativemedicine.arizona.edu/about/definition.html

9. Lahtz, Christoph and Gerd P. Pfeifer, 'Epigenetic changes of DNA repair genes in cancer', *Journal of Molecular Cell Biology*, February 2011; https://pubmed.ncbi.nlm.nih.gov/21278452/

10. Konjengbam, Nirmala, 'Lack of awareness responsible for low health insurance penetration', *Outlook Money*, 17 November 2019; https://www.outlookindia.com/outlookmoney/insurance/lack-of-awareness-responsible-for-low-health-insurance-penetration-3896

11. WHO, 'COVID-19: vulnerable and high-risk groups', accessed 24 January 2020; https://www.who.int/westernpacific/emergencies/covid-19/information/high-risk-groups

12. WHO, 'Cardiovascular diseases (CVDs)/Key facts', accessed 18 January 2021; https://www.who.int/en/news-room/fact-sheets/detail/cardiovascular-diseases-(cvds)

13. Newcastle University, 'Type 2 diabetes is a reversible condition', ScienceDaily, 13 September 2017.

14. D. Ornish et al., 'Intensive lifestyle changes for reversal of coronary heart disease', *JAMA*, 280 (23), 16 Dec 1998: 2001–07; doi: 10.1001/jama.280.23.2001; Erratum in: *JAMA*, 281 (15), 21 Apr. 1999:1380; PMID: 9863851; https://www.ncbi.nlm.nih.gov/pubmed/9863851

15. S. Wu et al., 'Substantial contribution of extrinsic risk factors to cancer development', *Nature*, 529, 2016: 43–47; https://doi.org/10.1038/nature16166; https://www.sciencedaily.com/releases/2020/02/200225143511.htm

16. Chhachhi, Rachna, *You Can Beat Cancer: Expert Advice on Preventing and Reversing Cancer*, Jaico Publishing House, 2020

17. Donaldson, Michael S., 'Nutrition and cancer: a review of the evidence for an anti-cancer diet', *Nutrition Journal*, 3 (19), 20 Oct. 2004; doi:10.1186/1475-2891-3-19

18. Paul V. Viscuse et al., 'Integrative medicine in cancer survivors', *Current Opinion in Oncology*, 29 (4), 2017: 235–42; doi:10.1097/CCO.0000000000000376

19. Linda Mah et al., 'Can anxiety damage the brain?', *Current Opinion in Psychiatry*, 29 (1), 2016: 56; doi: 10.1097/YCO.0000000000000223

20. Christopher Blank et al., 'Emotional Footprints of Email Interruptions', Proceedings of the 2020 CHI Conference on Human Factors in Computing Systems, Association for Computing Machinery, New York, NY, USA, 2020: 1–12; doi:https://doi.org/10.1145/3313831.3376282

21. The Healer's Journal, 'The 7 quantum physics theories that explain how everything is made of energy', accessed 18 January 2021; http://www.thehealersjournal.com/2013/05/05/quantum-physics-explain-how-everything-is-made-of-energy/

22. Jain, S. and P.J. Mills, 'Biofield Therapies: Helpful or Full of Hype? A Best Evidence Synthesis', *International Journal of Behavioral Medicine*, 2009; doi: 10.1007/s12529-009-9062-4

23. Antoine Louveau et al., 'Structural and functional features of central nervous system lymphatic vessels', *Nature*, 2015; doi: 10.1038/nature14432

24. Ivana Buric et al., 'What Is the Molecular Signature of Mind–Body Interventions? A Systematic Review of Gene Expression Changes Induced by Meditation and Related Practices', *Frontiers in Immunology*, 2017; 8 doi: 10.3389/fimmu.2017.00670 in Immunology, 2017; 8 DOI: 10.3389/fimmu.2017.00670

25. Kevin J. Miller, et al., 'Habits without Values', bioRxiv 067603; doi: https://doi.org/10.1101/067603

26. Christian Luis Bender et al., 'Emotional stress induces structural plasticity in Bergmann glial cells via an AC5-CPEB3-GluA1 pathway', *The Journal of Neuroscience*, 2020; JN-RM-0013-19; doi: 10.1523/JNEUROSCI.0013-19.2020

27. Toni-Lee Sterley et al., 'Social transmission and buffering of synaptic changes after stress', *Nature Neuroscience*, 2018; doi: 10.1038/s41593-017-0044-6

28. As explained in the restore Community Holistic Healthcoach Certification Program by faculty member, Dr Bhavana Gautam, emotional well-being specialist

29. WHO, 'Depression', accessed 18 January 2021; https://www.who.int/health-topics/depression#tab=tab_1

30. Anup Sharma et al., 'A Breathing-Based Meditation Intervention for Patients With Major Depressive Disorder Following Inadequate Response to Antidepressants', *The Journal of Clinical Psychiatry*, 2016; doi: 10.4088/JCP.16m10819

31. June C. Lo et al., 'Sleep Duration and Age-Related Changes in Brain Structure and Cognitive Performance', *SLEEP*, 2014; doi: 10.5665/sleep.3832

32. Van Cauter, E., 'Short sleep, poor sleep: novel risk factors for type 2 diabetes', *FASEB J*, 23, 2009: 417.4-417.4; https://doi.org/10.1096/fasebj.23.1_supplement.417.4

33. Max Hirshkowitz et al., 'National Sleep Foundation's sleep time duration recommendations: methodology and results summary', *Sleep Health* (Journal of the National Sleep Foundation), 2015; doi: 10.1016/j.sleh.2014.12.010

34. Leproult, Rachel and Eve V. Cauter, 'Role of Sleep and Sleep Loss in Hormonal Release and Metabolism', *Endocrine Reviews*, 24 November 2009; https://www.ncbi.nlm.nih.gov/pmc/articles/PMC3065172/

35. Eti Ben Simon et al., 'Overanxious and under slept', *Nature Human Behaviour*, 2019; doi: 10.1038/s41562-019-0754-8

36. Karine Spiegel et al., 'Impact of sleep debt on metabolic and endocrine function', 354, (9188), 23 October 1999: 1435–39; doi:https://doi.org/10.1016/S0140-6736(99)01376-8

37. Karine Spiegel et al., 'Sleep Curtailment in Healthy Young Men Is Associated with Decreased Leptin Levels, Elevated Ghrelin Levels, and Increased Hunger and Appetite', *Annals of Internal Medicine*, 7 December 2004; https://doi.org/10.7326/0003-4819-141-11-200412070-00008

38. Monika Eckstein et al., 'Oxytocin Facilitates the Extinction of Conditioned Fear in Humans', *Biological Psychiatry*, 2014; doi: 10.1016/j.biopsych.2014.10.015

39. You and Your Hormones, 'Oxytocin', accessed 18 January 2021; https://www.yourhormones.info/hormones/oxytocin/

40. Daisuke Yamada et al., 'Selective agonists of the δ-opioid receptor, KNT-127 and SNC80, act differentially on extinction learning of contextual fear memory in mice', *Neuropharmacology*, 2019; 160: 107792; doi: 10.1016/j.neuropharm.2019.107792

41. Hisayuki Amano et al., 'Telomere Dysfunction Induces Sirtuin Repression that Drives Telomere-Dependent Disease', *Cell Metabolism*, 2019; doi: 10.1016/j.cmet.2019.03.001

42. Linda E. Carlson et al., 'Mindfulness-based cancer recovery and supportive-expressive therapy maintain telomere length relative to controls in distressed breast cancer survivors', *Cancer*, 2014; doi: 10.1002/cncr.29063

43. Dean Ornish et al., 'Effect of comprehensive lifestyle changes on telomerase activity and telomere length in men with biopsy-proven low-risk prostate cancer: 5-year follow-up of a descriptive pilot study', *The Lancet Oncology*, 17 September 2013; doi: 10.1016/S1470-2045(13)70366-8

44. H. Lavretsky et al., 'A pilot study of yogic meditation for family dementia caregivers with depressive symptoms: effects on mental health, cognition, and telomerase activity', *International Journal of Geriatric Psychiatry*, 2012; doi: 10.1002/gps.3790

45. Loyola University Health System, 'When a broken heart becomes a real medical condition', ScienceDaily, 10 February 2015; www.sciencedaily.com/releases/2015/02/150210130502. htm

46. Sheldon Cohen et al., 'Chronic stress, glucocorticoid receptor resistance, inflammation, and disease risk', *PNAS*, 2 April 2012; doi: 10.1073/pnas.1118355109

47. Ibid.

48. James L. Oschman et al., 'The effects of grounding (earthing) on inflammation, the immune response, wound healing, and prevention and treatment of chronic inflammatory and autoimmune diseases', *Journal of Inflammation Research*, vol. 8, 24 Mar. 2015: 83–96; doi:10.2147/JIR.S69656https://www. ncbi.nlm.nih.gov/pmc/articles/PMC4378297/

49. J. Miguel Cisneros-Franco et al., 'A Brain without Brakes: reduced Inhibition Is Associated with Enhanced but Dysregulated Plasticity in the Aged Rat Auditory Cortex', *eNeuro*, 2018; ENEURO.0051-18.2018; doi: 10.1523/ ENEURO.0051-18.2018

50. Beavers, Kristen M., and Barbara J. Nicklas, 'Effects of lifestyle interventions on inflammatory markers in the metabolic syndrome', *Frontiers in bioscience* (Scholar edition), vol. 3, 1 Jan. 2011: 168–77; doi:10.2741/s142

51. Radha Goel et al., 'Exercise-Induced Hypertension, Endothelial Dysfunction, and Coronary Artery Disease in a Marathon Runner', *The American Journal of Cardiology*, 99 (5), 1 March 2007: 743–44; doi: https://doi.org/10.1016/j. amjcard.2006.09.127

52. Erin J. Howden et al., 'Reversing the Cardiac Effects of Sedentary Aging in Middle Age—A Randomized Controlled Trial: Implications For Heart Failure Prevention', *Circulation*, 2018; CIRCULATIONAHA.117.030617; doi: 10.1161/CIRCULATIONAHA.117.030617

53. The American College of Cardiology, 'Yoga and Aerobic Exercise Together May Improve Heart-Disease Risk Factors', 19 October 2017, accessed 24 January 2021; https://www.acc.org/about-acc/press-releases/2017/10/19/08/47/yoga-and-aerobic-exercise-together-may-improve-heart-disease-risk-factors

54. Tucker, Larry A., 'Physical activity and telomere length in U.S. men and women: An NHANES investigation', *Preventive Medicine*, 24 April 2007; https://pubmed.ncbi.nlm.nih.gov/28450121/

55. Ibid.

56. Institute of Medicine (US) Panel on Dietary Antioxidants and Related Compounds, 'Dietary Reference Intakes for Vitamin C, Vitamin E, Selenium, and Carotenoids. Washington (DC): National Academies Press (US); 2000. 2, Vitamin C, Vitamin E, Selenium, and β-Carotene and Other Carotenoids: Overview, Antioxidant Definition, and Relationship to Chronic Disease'; https://www.ncbi.nlm.nih.gov/books/NBK225471/https://www.ncbi.nlm.nih.gov/books/NBK225471/

57. Carmen Hurtado del Pozo et al., 'A Receptor of the Immunoglobulin Superfamily Regulates Adaptive Thermogenesis', *Cell Reports*, 28 (3), 2019: 773; doi: 10.1016/j.celrep.2019.06.061

58. India Today Web Desk, 'India is the most depressed country in the world. Here's a list of countries with the greatest burden of mental and behavioural disorders, in terms of most years of life lost due to disability or death adjusted for population size,

according to WHO', India Today, 1 November 2019; https://www.indiatoday.in/education-today/gk-current-affairs/story/india-is-the-most-depressed-country-in-the-world-mental-health-day-2018-1360096-2018-10-10

59. Shreshtha Malvia et. al., 'Epidemiology of breast cancer in Indian women', *Asia Pacific Journal of Clinical Oncology*, 9 February 2017; https://onlinelibrary.wiley.com/doi/full/10.1111/ajco.12661

60. N.A. Lund-Blix et al., 'Maternal and child gluten intake and association with type 1 diabetes: The Norwegian Mother and Child Cohort Study', *PLoS Med*, 17 (3); e1003032; https://doi.org/10.1371/journal.pmed.1003032

61. Alessandra Bordoni et al., 'Dairy products and inflammation: A review of the clinical evidence', *Critical Reviews in Food Science and Nutrition*, 13 August 2017; https://pubmed.ncbi.nlm.nih.gov/26287637/

62. Harvard T.H. Chan School of Public Health, 'Study sheds light on dairy fat and cardiovascular disease risk', The Nutrition Source, 25 October 2016; https://www.hsph.harvard.edu/nutritionsource/2016/10/25/dairy-fat-cardiovascular-disease-risk/

63. L.A. Ferrara et al., 'Olive oil and reduced need for antihypertensive medications', *Archives of Internal Medicine*, 27 March 2000; https://pubmed.ncbi.nlm.nih.gov/10737284/

64. Yamuna Manoharan et al., 'Curcumin: a Wonder Drug as a Preventive Measure for COVID19 Management', *Indian Journal of Clinical Biochemistry*, 17 June 2020; https://www.ncbi.nlm.nih.gov/pmc/articles/PMC7299138/

65. S. Banerjee et al., 'Ancient drug curcumin impedes 26S proteasome activity by direct inhibition of dual-specificity tyrosine-regulated kinase 2'. *Proc Natl Acad Sci USA*, 115 (32), 7 Aug. 2018: 8155–60; doi: 10.1073/pnas.1806797115; Epub 2018 Jul 9; PMID: 29987021; PMCID: PMC6094102

66. B. Banaszewska et al., 'Effects of Resveratrol on Polycystic Ovary Syndrome: A Double-blind, Randomized, Placebo-controlled Trial. J Clin Endocrinol Metab', 101 (11), 2016 November: 4322–28; doi: 10.1210/jc.2016-1858; Epub 2016 Oct 18; PMID: 27754722

67. The University of Alabama at Birmingham (UAB), 'Red Wine Compound Shown To Prevent Prostate Cancer', UAB News Content, 31 August 2007; https://www.uab.edu/newsarchive/38276-red-wine-compound-shown-to-prevent-prostate-cancer

68. C. Andrews et al., 'Resveratrol suppresses NTHi-induced inflammation via up-regulation of the negative regulator MyD88 short', Sci Rep 6 (34445), 2016; https://doi.org/10.1038/srep34445

69. M. L. Chen et al., 'Resveratrol Attenuates Trimethylamine-N-Oxide (TMAO)-Induced Atherosclerosis by Regulating TMAO Synthesis and Bile Acid Metabolism via Remodeling of the Gut Microbiota', mBio, 7 (2), 5 Apr. 2016: e02210-15; doi: 10.1128/mBio.02210-15; PMID: 27048804; PMCID: PMC4817264

70. 'Cancer-Fighting Roles of Intriguing Plant Compounds', Agricultural Research magazine, July 2010, https://agresearchmag.ars.usda.gov/2010/jul/plant

71. Caldwell, Emily, 'The Compound in the Mediterranean Diet that Makes Cancer Cells "Mortal"', Food Innovation Center, The Ohio State University, accessed on 24 January 2021; https://fic.osu.edu/news/news-archive/mediterranean-diet-mortal.html

72. B. Ruiz-Núñez et al., 'Higher Prevalence of "Low T3 Syndrome" in Patients With Chronic Fatigue Syndrome: A Case-Control Study,' Front Endocrinol (Lausanne), 9:97, 20 Mar. 2018; doi: 10.3389/fendo.2018.00097; PMID: 29615976; PMCID: PMC5869352

73. Christine F. Skibola et al., 'Brown Kelp Modulates Endocrine Hormones in Female Sprague-Dawley Rats and in Human Luteinized Granulosa Cells', *The Journal of Nutrition*, 135 (2), February 2005: 296–300; https://doi.org/10.1093/jn/135.2.296

74. Ghislain Moussavou et al., 'Anticancer effects of different seaweeds on human colon and breast cancers', *Marine Drugs*, 12 (9), 24 Sep. 2014: 4898–911; doi:10.3390/md12094898

75. American Journal of Medicine, 'Moderate Alcohol Consumption in Middle Age Can Lower Cardiac Risk', Elsevier, 7 March 2008; https://www.elsevier.com/about/press-releases/research-and-journals/moderate-alcohol-consumption-in-middle-age-can-lower-cardiac-risk

76. Ibid.